# A Manual of Oral Medicine
## *second edition*

## Fergal F Nally
MD   FDSRCS (Eng.)   FFDRCSI

Senior Lecturer in Oral Medicine, Institute of Dental
Surgery, University of London, and Head of
Department and Honorary Consultant in Oral
Medicine, Eastman Dental Hospital, London

## Deryck J Eggleston
MB   BS   FDSRCS (Eng.)   FRACDS

Department of Oral Medicine/Oral Surgery,
Perth Dental Hospital, Western Australia
Oral and Maxillo Facial Surgeon, Royal Perth
Hospital, Western Australia

Manchester University Press

© 1973, Copyright 1983 Fergal F Nally,
and Deryck J Eggleston

Published by
Manchester University Press
at Oxford Road, Manchester M13 9PL, UK
and at 51 Washington Street, Dover,
New Hampshire 03820, USA

1st Edition 1973
Revised and Reprinted 1976, 1978

2nd Edition 1983

*British Library cataloguing in publication data*

Nally, Fergal F.
    A manual of oral medicine. — 2nd ed.
    1. Mouth — Diseases
    I. Title    II. Eggleston, Deryck J.

    ISBN 0-7190-0945-6

*Library of Congress cataloguing in publication data*

Nally, Fergal F.
    A manual of oral medicine
    Includes index.
    1. Mouth — diseases — handbooks, manuals etc.
    2. Oral manifestations of general diseases —
    handbooks, manuals etc. I. Eggleston,
    Deryck J.    II. Title.
    (DNLM: 1. Mouth diseases — outlines. WU18 N172M)
    RC815.N33 1982    616.3′1    83-895

    ISBN 0-7190-0945-6

Printed in Hong Kong
by Wing King Tong Co. Ltd.

# A Manual of Oral Medicine

# Contents

# Contents

**Foreword** **by Sir Robert Bradlaw,** CBE DDSc FRCS FDSRCS
Emeritus Professor of oral Medicine, University of
London and Hon. Professor of Oral Pathology, Royal
College of Surgeons of England.

Oral medicine is extending in both scope and
complexity all the time; this derives necessarily from
increased understanding of the basic aetiology and
interrelations of disorder and disease. Indeed more
and more symptom complexes, hitherto regarded as
entities, have come to be recognized as an expression
of a simple basic pathology.

The contribution that this manual makes has to be
assessed with regard to its purpose, which is to
facilitate reference and revision for those for whom
wider reading has provided the requisite background.
It does not purport to replace more comprehensive
works, but succinct in form and direct in approach, it
should prove helpful, especially to the postgraduate
student for whom, no doubt, it is primarily intended
and should encourage a study of recent advances of
significance in our field.

Anatole France said that to digest knowledge we must
have an appetite for it; these pages may serve to whet
that appetite.

**Preface to the First Edition**   Oral medicine has now become a well recognized speciality and yet the number of works on the subject is comparatively small.

The purpose of this book is to outline, in clinical terms, the essential features of the more common conditions in this field. It is intended primarily for the final year undergraduate and postgraduate student preparing for examinations. However, because of the significant development of oral medicine in recent years it is hoped that medical and dental practitioners alike will find it a useful stimulus to further reading.

**Preface to the Second Edition**   This edition has been produced in response to certain changes which have occurred in oral medicine in recent years. The general arrangement of chapters has been altered to give a better flow; new chapters on cancer and precancer, psychiatric disorders in dentistry, and disorders of the tongue and abnormalities of taste are included and most other chapters have been rewritten and enlarged.

The purpose of this book is still to present, mainly in clinical terms, the essential features of the more common diseases encountered in this speciality. Because most of the current texts are extensive and usually intended for reference, this work gives an outline of oral medicine that final year undergraduate and postgraduate students preparing for examinations should find helpful. It is intended to be read in conjunction with other texts, reviews and original papers, so that it will provide a framework to which additional knowledge can be added.

**Acknowledgements**   The authors are indebted to Sir Robert Bradlaw for his continuous advice and encouragement.

It is a pleasure to dedicate this work to our wives, Anne and Dianne, for their constant support.

## Chapter 1    Introduction

**Oral Mucosa**    Tissues classified according to function:
*Lining* — Cheeks, vestibules and under tongue.
*Masticatory* — Hard palate and gingiva.
*Specialized* — Dorsal surface of the tongue. The lining
mucosa is usually thin, not keratinized and allows
considerable tissue mobility. The masticatory mucosa
is keratinized and is able to withstand moderate
trauma. The tongue is supplied with a large number of
gustatory receptors and contains lymphoid tissue.

*Colour*    Four factors contribute to the colour of the oral mucosa.
1. Thickness of the mucosa.
2. Presence of melanin in the mucosa.
3. Amount of blood flowing through the mucosa.
4. Quality of blood flowing through the mucosa.

**Diagnosis**    The stages leading to a definitive diagnosis include
history, examination and special tests.

*History*    Duration of lesion.
The presence or absence of pain.
Onset — sudden or gradual.
Progress — lesion continuously present or intermittent.
Associated phenomena — for example, tissue swelling,
bleeding, discharge and skin rash.
Past medical, dental, personal (including occupation)
and family histories.

*Examination*    *Extra oral.* Skin lesions should be noted, together with
cervical lymph gland enlargement.
*Intra oral.* Inspection of the mucosa will reveal the
site, shape, size and quality of the surface; whether the
lesion is on or beneath the mucosa, and the colour of
the lesion. Palpation will determine whether the lesion
is hard, firm or soft; whether the edge is well outlined
or ill-defined, and its mobility.

*Special tests*    The clinical diagnosis may be confirmed by one or
more of the following procedures:
1. Biopsy
2. Culture
3. Cytology
4. Haematology and serology
5. Biochemistry
6. Radiology
7. Immunology studies

*Chapter 2*  **Immunology and Oral Disease**

**Definition**   An autoimmune disease is caused by an alteration in the immunoresponsive tissues whereby they react with other body tissues.

**Significance**   The study of autoimmune diseases has lead to a better understanding of their underlying pathology. This in turn has allowed more accurate diagnosis, better management, and more effective treatment.

*Characteristics of an autoimmune disorder*

1. Presence of specific autoantibodies.
2. Presence of other autoimmune symptoms.
3. Altered globulin may be deposited in the lesion.
4. Mononuclear cell infiltration in the lesion.
5. Hypergammaglobulinaemia.
6. Favourable response with corticosteroids.
7. Favourable response with immunosuppressive agents.

**Types**   The mouth may be involved indirectly or directly in the autoimmune process. An indirect relationship will occur when lesions start elsewhere, for example in the thyroid, stomach or adrenal gland; at some stage of the illness the mouth can be affected. On the other hand, in direct involvement — as in pemphigoid and pemphigus — lesions start in the mouth and may (or may not) spread to other parts of the body at a later stage.

An increasing number of disorders are being recognized as autoimmune. A useful classification is:

1. *Organ Specific*. This implies that the antigen – antibody reaction takes place in one tissue and a narrow range of tissue specificity is usual. Examples include Hashimoto's thyroiditis, primary hypothyroidism, thyrotoxicosis, chronic athrophic gastritis and primary adrenal atrophy. Immunization with extracts of the relevant organ and Freund's adjuvant can produce analogues of some of these diseases in animals.

2. *Non-Organ Specific*. Diffuse changes are found in many tissues. Antibodies usually demonstrate a wide range of organ and species specificity. Rheumatoid arthritis and lupus erythematous are examples. These conditions have not been produced in animals, except that Freund's adjuvant arthritis in rats has some similarities to rheumatoid arthritis, but the rheumatoid factor cannot be demonstrated.

3. *Mixed*. Lesions of the mixed type do not fall into either of the above groups.

**Diagnosis**

1. Specific humoral or cell-bound antibody should be demonstrated in the laboratory.
2. Antigen should be identified and should induce humoral or cell bound antibody in animals.
3. Antigenic stimulation of the animal should lead to the disease.
4. Experimental disease should be capable of passive transfer with serum or cells. It should be remembered that these four points are absolute diagnostic criteria used in academic research. The clinician should attempt only to identify specific factors (usually antibodies) and correlate them with the results of other findings such as biopsy, radiology, haematology, biochemistry, hormone assay etc. before coming to a definitive diagnosis. Examples of disorders will be mentioned below and their relationship to oral findings should be borne in mind.

*Organ specific*

1. *Thyroid*. Two antigen – antibody reactions are recognized in thyroid disorders; colloid antigen and thyroid microsomes may be antigenic.
2. *Stomach*. Antibodies to gastric parietal cells and to intrinsic factor have been found. Antibody appears to attack the microsomes of the gastric parietal (oxyntic) cells. It is probably not related to the duration of anaemia but has been found in 20 per cent of patients with iron deficiency anaemia. It is occasionally found in healthy people. Antibody against intrinsic factor can be found in approximately 50 per cent of patients with pernicious (Addisonian) anaemia.
3. *Adrenal gland*. Antibodies reacting with the cytoplasm of cells in the adrenal cortex have been demonstrated in approximately 50 per cent of cases of primary adrenal atrophy.

*Nonorgan-specific*

1. *Rheumatoid arthritis*. The rheumatoid arthritis factor (RA factor) is thought to react with immuno-globulin G (IgG) in the presence of complement to produce agglutination. These insoluble RA – IgG complexes are deposited in affected joints. The RA factor is a macroglobulin (IgM) and is produced in the cytoplasm of plasma cells. During an acute attack of arthritis the complement level in synovial fluid falls, probably because it is gradually used up in the formation of the insoluble complexes. These complexes are then phagocytosed by white cells, releasing lyzozymal enzymes which cause further joint

damage. The temporomandibular joints are affected in approximately 35 per cent of patients with rheumatoid arthritis. In addition to progressive joint destruction, other lesions may develop including subcutaneous nodules, gangrenous skin ulcers, necrotizing arthritis, peripheral neuropathy and diffuse interstitial pulmonary fibrosis.

2. Systemic lupus erythematous (SLE). The essential immunological finding in systemic lupus erythematous appears to be antibodies to various nuclear factors. Three antinuclear factors (ANFs) are recognized viz, homogenous, nucleolar and speckled. The ANF may be found in discoid LE. The severity of the lesions may depend on the aggressiveness and selectivity of the antibodies. DNA has been shown in the serum of patients with SLE and the renal damage that can occur might be due to circulating DNA–antibody complexes.

**Mixed type**

*Sjögren's syndrome.* This syndrome is a good example of the mixed type because a wide spectrum of immunological abnormalities may be present, including antibodies to salivary epithelium, positive RA factor, positive antinuclear factor and occasionally LE cells.

There also appears to be a close association between this syndrome and other autoimmune disorders — for example, rheumatoid arthritis, scleroderma and thyroiditis.

**Oral aspects**

Autoimmune disorders may have an indirect or direct relationship to the oral cavity.

**Indirect Oral Autoimmune Diseases**

There are a considerable number of systemic autoimmune disorders and the mouth may become involved at some stage of the illness. These include:

1. *Pernicious anaemia.* Glossitis and oral candidiasis are common findings in patients with this disease.

2. *Myxoedema.* Dental caries, malocclusion, periodontal disease, delayed eruption of teeth and poor bone development may be found especially in young patients.

3. *Rheumatoid arthritis.* The temporomandibular joints are affected in approximately 35 per cent of patients with rheumatoid arthritis.

4. *Lupus erythematosus.* 'Butterfly' pigmentation on the face and white oral mucosal lesions are usual in the discoid form and a non-specific stomatitis in the systemic form.

5. *Hypoparathyroidism.* Dental hypoplasia and persistent candidosis are well recognized oral complications, especially in young patients.
6. *Sjögren's syndrome.* Xerostomia, xerophthalmia and oral candidiasis are usually present.
7. *Scleroderma.* The tongue, soft palate and cheeks may be partially immobilized, giving rise to limitation of opening, dysarthria and dysphagia.

**Direct Oral Autoimmune Disease**

At present there are three conditions that affect the oral mucosa:
1. *Aphthous ulceration.* Circulating antibodies to the cytoplasm of oral squamous epithelium have been demonstrated in patients with aphthous ulcers. The histological changes appear to be consistent with a delayed hypersensitivity reaction.
2. *Pemphigus.* Circulating antibodies to the intercellular cement substance of oral squamous epithelium have been found; the titre appears to be directly related to the severity of the disorder.
3. *Bullous pemphigoid.* Circulating antibodies to the basement membrane zone of squamous epithelium have been found in this condition.
4. *Mucous membrane pemphigoid.* Antibodies to the basement membrane of squamous epithelium have been found in this condition using the direct immuno-fluorescent technique.

## Chapter 3 Oral Ulceration

**Definition**

An ulcer is a break in the surface continuity of skin or mucous membrane.

**Diagnosis**

History, examination and special tests lead to a diagnosis. Knowledge of the number of ulcers, and their duration, site, shape, size, base, floor, edge and discharge, is important.

**Classification**

*Primary ulceration.* This implies that the surface break in mucosa is present from the initial stages of the lesion.
*Secondary ulceration.* Mucosal ulceration can be secondary to rupture of vesicular and bullous lesions.

**Primary Ulceration**

1. *Traumatic.* Three types of trauma are recognized: physical, chemical and psychiatric. Trauma is probably the commonest cause of oral ulceration and usually results from sharp teeth, poorly fitting dentures, toothbrushing, chemicals or drugs such as aspirin, or psychosomatic factors such as cheek biting. Psychiatric trauma is sometimes difficult to diagnose; when present it is known as stomatitis artefacta. Dermatitis artefacta may also be an additional feature. The histological features are non-specific, and healing usually occurs without scar formation.
2. *Infective.* Acute ulcerative gingivostomatitis is associated with Vincent's spirochaete and *Bacillus fusiformis*. Predisposing factors include poor oral hygiene and smoking, upper respiratory tract infections and nutritional deficiency. The diagnosis is usually made on the sudden onset of acute stomatitis and general debility; there is a characteristic ulcerative lesion initially confined to the gingiva and a distinct halitosis. The patient is acutely ill and, if the condition is untreated, extensive tissue destruction can occur. Where chronic malnutrition is endemic this infection can lead on to *Cancrum oris*. The diagnosis may be confirmed by smear and by the response to metronidazole or penicillin. Tuberculous ulceration of the oral mucosa is usually secondary to pulmonary tuberculosis. Infected sputum probably enters a mucosal tear and sets up the characteristic reaction. The ulcer is usually persistent, single and shows

undermined edges, thus indicating the horizontal spread of the organisms in the subepithelial lymphatic plexus. Biopsy is probably the best method to confirm the diagnosis and steps, including chest X-rays, must be taken to identify a primary lesion. 'Snail track' syphilitic ulceration may be found in the secondary stage and deep 'punched out' ulcers in the tertiary stage. However, if an atypical ulcer together with white lesions are found with nothing to account for them in the history, one should then consider the possibility of syphilis. The histological features show lymphocytic infiltration, obliterative endarteritis and periosteal new bone formation. However, the final diagnosis is made on positive serological findings. Other infections that may cause ulceration of the oral mucosa are actinomycosis, candidiasis and infectious mononucleosis.

3. *Neoplastic.* Squamous cell carcinoma is the commonest cause of malignant ulceration. The tongue is the usual intra-oral site followed by the floor of the mouth, alveolar mucosa, palate and buccal mucosa. In the early stages the disease may be relatively painless and unfortunately may go unrecognized until it is too late.

4. *Systemic conditions.* There are a number of general conditions that are closely associated with oral ulceration and include anaemia, agranulocytosis, lupus erythematosus, lichen planus and Crohn's disease.

5. *Aphthous ulceration.* Diagnosis should present no great difficulty. There will be a history of recurrent ulceration for more than three months. Several ulcers develop and take about fourteen days to heal. Each ulcer is surrounded by a large area of inflammation. They have been classified as:
i)   Minor aphthous ulceration
ii)  Major aphthous ulceration
iii) Ulceration and other lesions — Behcet's syndrome, Reiter's disease
iv)  Herpetiform ulceration

**Findings in Aphthous Ulceration**

A number of findings in minor, major and Behcet's syndrome suggest that aphthous ulceration may have an autoimmune basis.
1. Antibodies to cytoplasm of oral epithelium have been demonstrated.
2. Mononuclear cell infiltration and increased mast cell count in the lesion.
3. Favourable response to corticosteroids. Viral, hormonal and psychogenic factors have been also suggested.

There is some evidence that aphthous ulceration may be related to a deficiency of certain haematinics. In severe cases, therefore in addition to a full blood count, the plasma iron, total iron binding capacity and per cent saturation, plasma folate and vitamin B12 levels should be measured. A rise in the serum fibrinogen level is a useful confirmatory procedure in Behcet's syndrome.

*Behcet's syndrome*   Oral, ocular and genital lesions — poor prognosis.

*Reiter's disease*   Genital, oral, ocular lesions and arthritis — good prognosis.

**Secondary Ulceration**   Oral bullous lesions may be classified on histological grounds as follows:
1. Intra-epithelial bullous lesions
2. Sub-epithelial bullous lesions

**Intra-epithelial bullous lesions**   1. *Herpes simplex.* Primary herpes simplex stomatitis usually occurs two or three days after the onset of severe constitutional symptoms, and this is an important distinguishing feature from acute ulcerative gingivitis. At the time of presentation the oral mucosa may be extensively inflamed and a considerable number of small ulcers are apparent. The course of the disease may be described in four stages:
(1) Mucosal erythema
(2) Localized vesicles which last a few hours
(3) Ulceration which may last from ten to fourteen days
(4) healing without scar formation.

The diagnosis can be confirmed by culture of the virus, cytological identification of the inclusion bodies of Lipschütz and a rising titre against the herpes simplex virus. The serological titre estimation is the most dependable diagnostic aid, but unfortunately, two blood samples taken at a two-week interval are necessary and so the result will not be available until the patient has recovered. Once the clinical manifestations have disappeared the virus probably remains at the primary site indefinitely and could account for milder recurrent attacks, e.g. herpes labialis.

Also, we should regard herpes labialis as an important occupational hazard in dentistry; immunity appears to have dropped by approximately 50 per cent in the adult population in London since the late 1940s. A herpetic whitlow is only a local manifestation in the dentist of what is usually a severe generalized illness which may rarely be fatal.

2. *Herpes zoster.* An acute viral infection of the extramedullary cranial nerve ganglia or posterior horn cells which is accompanied by skin and mucosal lesions. In most cases severe pain occurs followed by the characteristic unilateral peripheral eruption. If the trigeminal nerve is involved the forehead, cheek, chin and oral mucosa on one side may show lesions. The diagnosis can be confirmed by culture although this may be difficult as the virus exhibits a high degree of host specificity. Cytological identification of multi-nucleated giant cells and eosinophilic inclusion bodies are more easily identified than in herpes simplex infection. A rising titre to the herpes zoster virus is the most dependable diagnostic aid but this test has the same limitations as in herpes simplex.

3. *Herpangina.* This is a specific stomatitis and pharyngitis caused by one of the Coxackie group A viruses. It most frequently effects children and may occur in epidemic form. constitutional features are mild, and a sore throat is the usual clinical feature. Examination will reveal multiple ulcers on the soft palate, anterior pillars of the fauces and sometimes on the tongue.

The illness may last up to five days. Culture, cytological and serological tests are not routinely undertaken because of the transient nature of the illness.

4. *Hand, foot and mouth disease.* Hand, foot and mouth disease is due to one of the Group A Coxsackie viruses. It is a highly infectious condition which tends to occur in epidemics, affecting children more than adults. Painful vesicles occur on the soles of the feet and palms of the hands, and oral ulcers develop in every case.

5. *Foot and mouth disease.* This condition, which occurs in cattle, is a very rare infection in humans and can occur by eating contaminated food or by contact with infected animals. In humans, the incubation period is between two and eighteen days, after which vesicles occur in the mouth, throat and lips and there is salivation and pyrexia. Painful vesicles are also found on the palms, soles and interdigital spaces. They soon rupture and leave ulcers which heal without scarring within two weeks. Specific antibody can be detected on serological examination but there is no curative treatment. Hyperimmune serum for vaccination of humans or animals is only effective for about six months.

6. *Pemphigus vulgaris.* This is a rare disorder which exhibits bullae and erosions of skin and mucous membrane, acantholytic changes in epithelial cells, circulating antibodies in blood and, if untreated, a high mortality rate. The disease usually occurs in patients over the age of 40 years who often present with oral bullae and ulceration. The surrounding mucosa is relatively normal and a positive Nikolsky sign is common. In the initial stages the patient is remarkably free of any constitutional upset. The onset is usually slow and insidious — but progressive. After a variable period from two months to two years the skin may become involved. The larynx, pharynx, nasal mucosa, conjunctiva and anus may also be affected. The diagnosis is confirmed by biopsy, acantholytic cells on scrapings, and by demonstrating antibody to the intercellular substance of squamous epithelium. The intercellular epithelial antibody, which is found in the patient's serum, appears to rise in proportion to the extent of the illness and will fall again when the patient responds to treatment. It is therefore not only an important diagnostic test but also a dependable therapeutic index. The condition is treated with systemic corticosteroids and sometimes supplemented with immunosuppressive agents such as azathioprine which has a steroid-sparing affect.

7. *Familial benign chronic pemphigus.* This appears to be a much less aggressive form of pemphigus. Repeated attacks of bullae and erosions occur in the same part of the mouth and no constitutional upset is noted. The bullae are intraepithelial and partially acantholytic cells may be found. No circulating antibodies to squamous epithelium have been detected.

**Subepithelial bullous lesions**

1. *Erythema multiforme.* This condition occurs most frequently in young people and consists of recurrent attacks of a severe exfoliative stomatitis which may be accompanied by a dermatitis. The stomatitis is generalized and painful and severe secondary infection is usual. Haemorrhagic crusting of the lips and blood-filled bullae may be found. The skin lesions take the form of circular erythematous macules, papules and bullae on the hands and arms, feet and legs. Each attack lasts from two or three weeks which may be followed by a remission of about six months. Recurrence over some years is usual. The cause is obscure, although drug hypersensitivity and bacterial and viral infections are suggested factors. The mycoplasma organism and the herpes simplex virus

have been specifically incriminated in some cases. The diagnosis is essentially clinical and laboratory tests can only help to exclude other conditions.

2. *Benign mucous membrane pemphigoid.* This condition usually presents in elderly people and is a bullous disorder that primarily involves the mouth. The eyes, vagina and rectum are sometimes affected. The onset is gradual and bullae are smaller and stronger than in pemphigus vulgaris. The surrounding mucosa is erythematous. Eventually, the bullae collapse and leave a painful ulcerated area partially covered by white tags of epithelium. The diagnosis is confirmed by the presence of a subepithelial bulla. Patients may have antibodies to the basement membrane zone of epithelium. This is usually found by the direct immunofluorescent test; a biopsy of the patient's mucosa is used in addition to a blood sample. Occasionally, the indirect test is positive on blood samples alone, but the titre is not always proportional to the severity of the disease.

3. *Bullous and erosive lichen planus.* Bullous lichen planus is a rare condition in the mouth. The diagnosis can be confirmed by the presence of the characteristic skin lesions on the flexor surfaces, the various striated mucosal patterns in addition to the erosions, absence of ocular involvement and the typical histological appearances of lichen planus.

4. *Epidermolysis bullosa.* This is a rare condition, usually affecting children, and may occur in the mouth. Bullae can be produced by minimal friction and a positive Nikolsky sign is usual. The oral findings may be associated with dystrophic skin changes.

In the severe form the mortality rate is considerable. The diagnosis is made on a long history of bullae caused by friction, dystrophic skin changes, a subepithelial bulla on biopsy, absence of acantholytic cells on cytology and absence of circulating antibodies to intercellular substance or basement membrane of squamous epithelium.

5. *Bullous pemphigoid.* This condition is primarily a skin disorder and rarely affects the mouth.

# Chapter 4  Cancer and Precancer

**Introduction**

Cancer of the mouth should concern dentists, doctors and patients because there appears to be a disturbingly high death rate in many countries. It is known that, in the United Kingdom, about 60 per cent of patients with cancer of the mouth die from it. The mutilation and disfigurement in those who survive can have devastating effects on patients and relatives. This poor outlook is regrettable because access to the mouth is so easy for examination, biopsy and early effective treatment. When discussing preventive measures the diagnosis and management of precancer should be considered.

**Epidemiology**

The relative frequency of oral cancer as a percentage of all cancers varies between 2 to 4 per cent in Europe and North America. In India it is as high as 40 per cent. In England and Wales there is a 10 per cent death rate within 5 years of diagnosis from lip cancer, 75 per cent from the tongue, 50 per cent from other regions of the mouth and 70 per cent from the oropharynx. This represents a total death rate of 60 per cent.

Squamous cell carcinoma accounts for 90 per cent of all oral cancers. The remaining 10 per cent includes adenocarcinoma, sarcoma and melanoma.

The main consideration of this chapter will be squamous cell carcinoma.

**Predisposing Factors**

Predisposition to oral carcinoma appears to come from two sources, (a) the precancerous oral lesion, and (b) the conditioning of the patient. Leukoplakia and erythroplakia have been regarded for many years as precancerous. Leukoplakia has been defined by the World Health Organization as 'a white patch or plaque that cannot be characterized clinically or pathologically as any other disease' and erythroplakia as 'a bright-red velvety plaque which cannot be characterized clinically or pathologically as being due to any other condition'.

The patient may be shown to have an underlying disease such as syphilis, reduced resistance to *Candida albicans*, chronic iron deficiency, oral submucous fibrosis or lichen planus. If an associated aetiology is known it is probably better to use such terms as syphilitic or candidal leukoplakia.

*Sublingual keratosis*
Leukoplakia or keratosis confined to the floor of the mouth and sublingual region was regarded until recently as a type of naevus. However, it is now thought not to be developmental and harmless, but definitely precancerous.

A painless soft white lesion under the tongue is usually found on routine examination. The surrounding mucosa is normal and gentle friction will not remove the lesion. Biopsy shows characteristic changes.

There appears to be a high risk of malignant transformation in sublingual keratosis. One estimate puts it at approximately 50 per cent, and malignancy in this area has a bad prognosis.

*Trauma*
Chronic irritation will probably produce a productive reaction in the oral mucosa. The common causes are friction, tobacco and alcohol. Chronic oral sepsis may also play a role. Onset is associated with physical or chemical factors.

**Clinical Types**
1. *Frictional keratosis.* This is commonly seen on the cheeks, tongue and commisures.
2. *Smoker's keratosis.* A definite pattern exists according to whether the patient smokes cigarettes, cigars, or a pipe. Cigarette smoking causes maximum keratosis in areas where saliva pools, for example on the lower part of the cheeks and lower vestibules. Lesions may also be noted on the dorsum of the tongue, commissures and lips. Pipe smoking will cause hyperkeratosis of the anterior hard palate, stomatitis nicotina on the posterior hard palate and erythema on the soft palate. Cigar smoking produces its maximum effect on the gingival tissues. Patients who consume snuff by mouth produce white lesions and pigmentation at the site of contact. This is usually inside the lower lip.
3. *Alcohol keratosis.* Excessive consumption of spirits may produce keratosis in the lower cheek mucosa.
4. *Chemical keratosis.* Chemicals may also produce white lesions, e.g. aspirin of phenol burns.

*Infection*
1. *Candidiasis.* The acute lesions caused by *Candida albicans* can be scraped gently from the mucosa and the diagnosis confirmed by culture on Sabouraud's medium. Serum and salivary antibodies can be measured. Chronic oral candidiasis may be an initial finding in other diseases, for example,

diabetes mellitus, anaemia and nutritional deficiencies.

There also appears to be a relationship in some cases with a multiple endocrinal deficiency state; and recent evidence suggests association between candidiasis and carcinoma.

In chronic oral candidiasis (candidal leukoplakia) the organisms invade the epithelium and produce hyperplasia. It is uncertain whether the organisms are the primary cause of the lesion or are only secondary invaders; but there is increasing evidence that they are the primary cause. There is a high risk of malignant change if the candidal leukoplakia remains, but it is not possible to assess the risk accurately.

2. *Syphilis.* Although chancres, mucous patches and gummas are well recognized lesions, generalized mucosal keratosis producing diffuse white patches are also found, especially in untreated patients. The reason for this is unknown and no *Treponema pallidum* organisms have been found in the keratotic areas.

The risk of carcinomatous degeneration in untreated syphilitic leukoplakia of the tongue appears to be high.

*Anaemia*

In long standing anaemia, especially due to iron deficiency, the oral mucosa tends to become atrophic. This may be further complicated by leukoplakia. In one series of patients with the Paterson-Kelly syndrome (also known as Plummer-Vinson) 18 per cent were found to have oral cancer.

*Lichen planus*

The mouth is often involved in lichen planus and sometimes the oral mucosa may be the only area affected. The cause is unknown. The diagnosis is usually made on a history of oral ulceration, the detection of white striae on the mucosa, and the histological appearance. Linear, papular, reticular, pigmented and erosive mucosal patterns have been described. Occasionally, subepithelial bullae may also be found. A skin eruption may be present. Trauma and emotional stress may be aggravating factors.

Reports of malignant change vary from one to 10 per cent in oral lichen planus.

**Management of Precancer**

Oral leukoplakia should be removed if it is compatible with good surgery. This is usually possible in well localized lesions but becomes more difficult in widespread involvement. Cryotherapy has been used with apparent short term success.

Attempts to remove mechanical trauma, and fungal infection should be made, underlying anaemia corrected and the patient asked to abstain from alcohol and tobacco. Oral lichen planus can be helped with topical corticosteroids.

Patients should be examined every three to six months, repeat biopsies undertaken where necessary.

## Chapter 5 Treatment of Oral Malignant Disease

Cancer patients ideally should be managed at a cancer centre. Specific treatment entails the use of surgery, radiotherapy, chemotherapeutic and hormonal agents. Hormones are not used in oral cancer and chemotherapeutic agents are used only for palliation. A joint decision by the surgeon and radiotherapist determines the best therapy in each case. If there is an equal choice between surgery and radiotherapy the latter is preferred as it avoids disfigurement.

### Radiotherapy

*Ionizing radiation*

Produced by X-ray generators, radium, and radioactive isotopes.
1. *Corpuscular.* Alpha rays have a poor tissue penetration not suitable for radiotherapy. Beta rays are sometimes used for superficial radiotherapy.
2. *Electromagnetic.* Gamma rays have deep tissue penetration. They are widely used and are the same as X-rays. X-rays are produced in generators. The energy of each radiation is described in electronvolts (eV). The higher the generating voltage the greater the penetration.

| Voltage | Range of generating energy |
|---|---|
| Low or superficial X-rays. | 10000 – 80000 eV (or 10 – 80 kilovolts (kv)). |
| Orthovoltage ('Deep X-rays'). | 80 – 400 kv. |
| Mega voltage. | above 1 million electronvolts (MeV). |

Mega electronvoltage (MeV) is the most efficient means of irradiating oral cancer, but many treatment centres only possess orthovoltage equipment. The Van de Graaff generator produces mega voltage energy up to 2 MeV. This machine is not as efficient as the linear accelerator which produces energy for therapeutic purposes of 4 – 6 MeV.

*Advantages of mega-voltage radiation*

1. *Greater penetration.* (Hence greater depth dose.)
2. *'Skin sparing' effect.* The dose to the skin is reduced because the maximum ionization occurs below skin surface.

The limiting factor with orthovoltage is the skin reaction.

3. *'Bone sparing' effect*. Differences between hard and soft tissues become unimportant. With lower energy X-rays, bone absorbs more of the rays and becomes prone to osteoradionecrosis.

4. *Minimal scatter*. The beam travels accurately in a straight line and incidental radiation is small, e.g. it is usually possible to preserve some parotid function by accurate alignment. Mega volt energy is also produced by gamma radiation from certain radioactive materials, e.g. radium and cobalt 60 (1 – 3 MeV).

Provided that the tumour is being correctly irradiated and the surrounding tissues spared, the source of the mega radiations is of minor importance.

*Radioactive materials*     Radium is most widely used. It gives off alpha, beta and gamma rays, but only the gamma rays are utilized. Cobalt 60 and caesium 137 are isotopes used as substitutes.

*Surface applicators*     Used in the treatment of some superficial tumours of the buccal mucosa, floor of the mouth or antral cavity. Isotopes are carried to the tumour area on a removable dental appliance.

*Implantation*     Radioactive materials are implanted in accessible tumours of the buccal mucosa or floor of the mouth. The implants are removed after about seven days.

*Radiation absorbed dose*     *Rad* (radiation absorbed dose) is the measure of radiation absorption and is the measure of all types of ionizing radiation. It is a unit of more practical value than the roentgen which is the unit of radiation exposure and used only for gamma and X-ray radiation.

**Oral Complications of Radiotherapy**     Complications tend to be mild but are worse with orthovoltage therapy. Full blood counts are a routine during treatment to guard against bone marrow depression.

*Skin*. Depigmentation, telangiectasis or atrophy may occur with orthovoltage.

*Mucositis*. Desquamation of the mucosa always occurs to some extent, but is usually temporary.

*Xerostomia*. Decreased salivary flow is the commonest persistent complication. It is more common with orthovoltage and isotope treatment.

*Dental caries*. The characteristic sites are the cervical margins; the condition probably relates to altered salivary function. Extensive conservation work is strongly recommended in order to avoid the need for extraction.

*Bone.* Osteoradionecrosis is rare, but the blood supply to the bone becomes reduced as endarteritis develops. Trauma to the jaws (e.g. extractions) after radiotherapy may cause osteoradionecrosis to spread; hence all dental sepsis must be eradicated before radiotherapy.

**Tooth Extraction**

*Orthovoltage.* Teeth in the treatment field must be extracted prior to radiotherapy regardless of their condition, to prevent osteoradionecrosis of the bone at a later stage.

*Mega voltage.* Teeth which are heavily filled or unsound must be extracted prior to treatment. Healthy teeth may be left even if they lie in the treatment beam.

*Applicators and Implants.* Teeth lying adjacent to the tumour must be removed prior to treatment even if they are healthy.

*Extractions during or after treatment.* If it is necessary to extract during treatment do so before the maximum dose is delivered or wait at least four weeks after treatment is finished. Endarteritis commences at six months and all extractions after this period should be performed in hospital with full antibiotic cover.

**Surgery**

*Indications for surgery in oral cancer:*
1. Small accessible lesions, provided that surgery does not produce multilation, e.g. wedge resection of tongue tip.
2. Tumours involving bone. The response to radiotherapy is poor with these tumours.
3. Radioresistant tumours.
4. Recurrences of tumours after a satisfactory regression has followed a course of radiotherapy.
5. Lymph node metastasis. Mobile nodes and well differentiated tumours are best treated by block dissection. Fixed nodes are inoperable. Lymph node metastasis from primitive tumours require radiotherapy.
6. 'Leukoplakia.' The malignancy may respond to radiotherapy but in some cases the area of leukoplakia recurs. Surgical stripping and skin grafting are required.

**Chemotherapy**

Chemotherapies treatment of choice of widespread disease. Several groups of drugs influence neoplastic stem cells. Their use in oral cancer is limited to palliation.

1. *Alkylating agents.* Their activity is due to the ability of the alkyl radical to combine with deoxyribonucleic acid (DNA) and cause major disturbances in cell replication. Alkylating agents include nitrogen mustard, chlorambucil, cyclophosphamide.

2. *Antimetabolites.* These act by competing with enzymes and blocking metabolic pathways involved with nucleic acid synthesis.

i) *Folic acid antagonists.* Methotrexate is the only folic acid antagonist in clinical use and is the most effective drug used in head and neck cancer. If used prior to surgery or radiotherapy, it may reduce tumour bulk. It is given systemically; intra-arterial infusion has been discarded.

ii) *Purine and pyrimidine antagonists* are not used in head and neck cancer. This group of drugs include mercaptopurine, azathioprine, cytosine, arabinoside.

3. *Plant alkaloids.* These agents arrest cell division in metaphase. The principal agents are vincristine and vinblastine, both of which are derived from the West Indian periwinkle plant.

4. *Antibiotics.* These antineoplastic drugs are derived from various species of the fungus *Streptomyces*, e.g. daunorubicin, actinomycin D and bleomycin. Bleomycin is useful in head and neck cancer. It is given intramuscularly or intravenously.

5. *Miscellaneous.* This group includes drugs with unique mechanism of action such as enzyme inhibition. L-asparaginase breaks down asparagine, depriving neoplastic cells of the enzyme which they are unable to synthesize themselves. Procarbazine inhibits nuclear acid synthesis by a mechanism not yet understood.

**Toxic Effects** Toxic effects are common and are usually dose-related. Bone marrow depression and gastrointestinal disturbance occur to some extent with all therapeutic agents. The latter presents as nausea, vomiting, severe ulcerative stomatitis and enteritis. Oral ulceration may also reflect the low white cell count or a fixed drug reaction.

**Cancer and Immunity** Efforts to stimulate immune function in patients with malignant disease have been equivocal. Specific therapy with inactivated tumour cells (vaccine) have produced conflicting results. Greater success has been claimed for non-specific methods of stimulating the immune system. BCG has been used widely, particularly for skin cancers, and the drug levamisole is used for controlling breast and lung cancer. Although there are many immunotherapy trials in progress, there are few which have shown therapeutic benefit over the longer term. An additional problem is that some of these agents may stimulate the growth of a tumour rather than destroy it.

## Chapter 6 Facial Pain

**Pain Afferent System**
Sensory fibres from facial structures are conveyed centrally in the trigeminal, facial and glossopharyngeal nerves as well as in afferents from the cervical 2 and 3 segments.
Impulses reach the thalamus and are relayed bilaterally to four important areas:
1. *Hypothalamus*. The autonomic responses to pain, including respiratory, cardiovascular and endocrinal, occur in the hypothalamic region.
2. *Temporal cortex*. The memory response to previous pain appears to be stored in the temporal cortex.
3. *Sensory cortex*. The nature and site of facial pain is perceived in the sensory cortex.
4. *Frontal cortex*. The emotional response to pain arises in the orbital part of the frontal lobe.

**Diagnosis**
Diagnosis may be difficult, especially in the absence of physical signs. However, the history, examination and special tests usually lead to a definitive diagnosis.

**History**
The history must include the following information:
1. *Site*. The patient should point with one finger to the area of maximum severity.
2. *Type*. The nature of the pain, whether sharp or dull, should be determined.
3. *Periodicity*. The relation to time, whether intermittent or continuous, should be recorded.
4. *Duration*. If intermittent, the duration of each attack is noted.
5. *Radiation*. Spread of pain to other areas.
6. *Provoking factors*. Thermal changes, eating, yawning, or lightly touching the face can all provoke pain.
7. *Relieving factors*. Heat, pressure or analgesics.
8. *Associated phenomena*. Swelling, bleeding and bad taste, may have been noticed by the patient.

**Aetiology**
The commonest causes of facial pain are dental and temporomandibular joint disturbances.

*Oral conditions*
Common oral lesions include pulpitis, stomatitis, periodontitis and osteitis. It has been shown that by electrically stimulating dental pulp pain may be experienced in remote parts of the face. After the

stimulus is removed facial pain still persists and at a time when no pulpal pain is felt.

*Temporomandibular joint lesions*

Perhaps the commonest cause of pain arising in the temporomandibular joint is minor trauma and about 80 per cent of cases are associated with poor or deficient occlusion of teeth.

*Ears, nose and throat conditions*

A large number of conditions in the nose, throat and ears may be responsible for facial pain. If a patient complains of deafness, tinnitus and tenderness in the mastoid region together with facial pain, an auricular lesion should be suspected. An unusual cause is nasopharyngeal carcinoma (Trotter's syndrome).

*Ocular conditions*

Corneal ulceration, iritis and glaucoma may be obvious causes on examination. However, it is always wise to keep in mind the possibility of a cerebellopontine angle tumour as an underlying cause of facial pain, and the corneal reflex should be elicited.

*Salivary gland lesions*

Well known lesions include suppurative parotitis, mumps and salivary calculi.

*Causalgia*

Causalgia is a rather ill-defined condition in which pain persists after trauma. Its nature is uncertain but is probably central in origin.

*Nerve lesions*

a) Paroxysmal trigeminal neuralgia.
b) Paroxysmal glossopharyngeal neuralgia.
Paroxysmal neuralgia of the fifth or ninth cranial nerves is of unknown aetiology. The diagnosis is usually made on the characteristic history of intermittent paroxysms of acute lancinating pain of short duration with complete freedom from pain between attacks. There are no significant clinical findings except a trigger area and a total lack of positive findings from special investigations. The pain is relieved by diagnostic block injection of local anaesthetic and there is a good response to a therapeutic trial of carbamazepine. Open nerve freezing by cryotherapy has been shown to be effective in both mild and severe cases.
c) Lesions involving the ganglia include herpes zoster and post herpetic neuralgia.

*Vascular*

a) *Migraine*. The underlying cause is believed to be related to vascular instability of the cerebral vessels. The incidence is 10 per cent in the general population, and 75 per cent of patients are women, many of whom are under 20 years of age. Premonitory sensations are visual, olfactory, gustatory and auditory and may be due to initial selective vasoconstriction of cerebral vessels. These are followed by pain whose distribution is constant for a particular patient; the frontal area seems to be the most common site.

b) *Periodic migrainous neuralgia.* This is more common in men, usually aged between 20 – 40 years. Pain occurs at regular intervals and is sited unilaterally under the eye. It is associated with epiphora, redness of the eye, nasal blockage and erythema of the skin on the same side. The patient may have an obsessional type of personality.

c) *Temporal arteritis.*

*Referred pain*  Pain may be referred to the facial structures from many areas which include:

i) *Heart.* Pain may be referred to the left angle of the mandible in a patient suffering from coronary sclerosis or thrombosis. Cervical sympathetic nerve fibres probably convey pain impulses to the thalamus.

ii) *Cervical intervertebral disc.* A prolapsed disc in cervical 2 and 3 region may also give rise to pain at the angle of the mandible by pressing on nerve fibres between the vertebrae.

*Atypical facial pain*  Pain of psychogenic origin. This is not a well known condition and a diagnosis is usually made by exclusion of all organic causes. It is more common in women and the pattern of pain distribution may be anatomically bizarre. A number of predisposing factors have been suggested and include endogenous and reactive depression, obsessional neurosis and hysteria.

*Significance*  Facial pain may be insignificant or a death sentence, depending on the aetiology. The patient's reaction will depend on whether the cause is known to him, its severity, location and its psychological predisposition.

## Chapter 7    Sensory and Motor Disorders of the Face

**Sensory Disorders**    Numbness or parasthesia in the face indicates a disturbance of the trigeminal nerve. The symptoms may be associated with impaired motor function. Concurrent cranial nerve signs are suggestive of a serious neurological disorder.

**Anatomy of the Trigeminal Nerve**    The central nuclei of both motor and sensory components are found in the pons. The central sensory ramifications spread to the cortex, midbrain, medulla and spinal cord.
Motor and sensory roots cross the cerebellopontine angle in the posterior cranial fossae after leaving the pons. The sensory root expands to form the trigeminal (gasserian) ganglion which contains the sensory relays of the nerve. The mandibular (3rd) division is joined by the motor root in the infratemporal fossa, but the 1st and 2nd division have no motor component. All forms of sensation must pass to the gasserian ganglion sensory root and the brain stem.

**Tests of Trigeminal Nerve Function**    *Sensory function.* Altered responses to pinprick, light touch and temperature should be noted.
*Motor function.* The temporalis and masseter muscles are assessed by palpation. Weakness in the pterygoid muscles may be detected by opening the mouth against resistance.
*Corneal reflex.* Touching the cornea with a piece of cotton wool normally produces bilateral blinking of the eyes. Loss of this reflex is often the first sign of trigeminal nerve disease.

**Aetiology**    The most important task is to exclude an underlying neoplasm.

**Peripheral Lesions**    Dental disease accounts for a high proportion of cases of peripheral lesions.
*Dental procedures*
(a) Surgical extraction of posterior mandibular teeth (particularly 3rd molars).
(b) Direct trauma to the nerves following local anaesthetic injections, osteotomy procedures or careless flap retraction.

*Infections*
(a) Acute abscess on lower posterior teeth or upper lateral incisors.
(b) Infected haematoma following a local anaesthetic.
(c) Osteomyelitis of the mandible.
(d) Infected cysts.

*Fractures*
(a) Fracture of body of the mandible behind the mental foramen.
(b) Fracture of the middle 3rd of the face.
(c) Fracture of condyle is a rare cause.
(d) Fracture of base of skull — an uncommon injury.

*Neoplasms*
Malignant tumours produce anaesthesia by direct invasion of nerves; examples include carcinoma of the buccal mucosa, antral neoplasms and secondary deposits. Nasopharyngeal carcinoma is particularly important as the close proximity of the basal skull foramina to the nasopharynx allows early invasion of the maxillary and mandibular branch of the Vth nerve. Over half the patients with nasopharyngeal carcinoma first present with neurological signs and most of these cases exhibit facial numbness and deafness.

**Central Lesions**   Neoplasms
(a) *Intrinsic*. A neurinoma arising directly from the nerve sheath or gasserian ganglion causes complete trigeminal anaesthesia.
(b) *Extrinsic*. Neoplasms arising in the cerebellopontine angle produce clinical features by compression. Tumours include acoustic neuromas (70%), Meningiomas (6%) and gliomas (6%). Loss of the corneal reflex may be the first sign of a cerebellopontine angle tumour.
(c) *Metastatic*. Deposits may involve the trigeminal nerve anywhere from the pons to the skin.
(d) *Neuropathic*. Gross sensory abnormalities can occur in cancer patients without any secondary deposits being found. Carcinoma of the lung is most commonly associated with this disturbance.

*Trauma (iatrogenic)*
Injection of alcohol into the gasserian ganglion or section of the sensory root of the trigeminal nerve have been used as treatment for intractable trigeminal neuralgia.

Vascular
(a) *Thrombosis*. Occlusion of the vessel supplying the lateral portion of the medulla causes facial

anaesthesia, Horner's syndrome, ataxia, and weakness of the tongue. Facial anaesthesia persists after the other signs regress.

(b) *Aneurysms.* These may act as space occupying lesions in the cerebellopontine angle or in the cavernous sinus region.

*Benign Trigeminal Sensory Neuropathy*
This is a transient numbness of one or more divisions of the trigeminal nerve. The aetiology is unknown but it seldom occurs until the second decade. The corneal reflex is not affected. The benign nature of the condition can only be confirmed by the passage of time.

*Infection*
(a) *Acute.* Middle ear infection may spread to the apex of the petrous bone involving the Vth and VIth nerves (Gradenigo's syndrome).

**Bell's Palsy**

*Aetiology.* Unknown. Probably oedema produces ischaemia of the nerve while in the facial canal.
Clinical features. Rapid, painful onset. Taste may be affected and transient deafness produced. Pain is localized around the ear.
Prognosis. Good, but persistent paralysis occurs in 10 per cent of cases.
Treatment. Analgesics for pain, protection for the patient's eyes and systemic corticosteroids.

**Other Causes of Lower Motor Neurone Paralysis**

1. *Cerebellopontine angle lesions.* (Paralysis is often bilateral). Neoplasms (acoustic neuroma, meningioma). Basal meningitis, aneurysm, fracture of base of skull and Guillaine-Barré syndrome.
2. *Choleastoma.* 80 per cent have facial palsy often associated with discharging ears and hearing loss.
3. *Lesions of facial canal.* Chronic middle ear infections, sarcoidosis, head injury and severe hypertension.
4. *Peripheral lesions.* (Often produce incomplete paralysis.) Salivary gland neoplasms, parotid surgery, stab wounds and birth injury caused by obstetric forceps.

**Bilateral Facial Paralysis**

*Muscle disorders.* Myasthenia gravis and Dystrophia myotonica.

*Nerve lesions.* Sarcoidosis, leprosy, Guillaine-Barré syndrome and chronic basal meningitis.

**Recommendations**　(1) a full neurological examination is required. Look particularly for V, VI and VII nerve signs.
(2) Test for hearing loss and look for discharge and other signs of middle ear disease.
(b) *Chronic*. Results in a thickened tough adherent membrane over the base of the brain. The meninges may be involved (syphilis) or an exudate formed (tuberculosis).
*Miscellaneous causes.*
Drugs, collagen disorders, hysteria, multiple sclerosis and syringobulbia.

**Complications of Trigeminal Sensory Loss**　Trigeminal sensory loss is uncommon. It usually occurs after the surgical treatment of trigeminal neuralgia or following vascular lesions of the brain stem.
(a) *Herpes simplex*. Blisters or sores appear within three days after the onset of anaesthesia.
(b) *Eye*. Decreased corneal sensitivity and failure of tear secretion lead to keratitis, conjunctivitis and iritis.
(c) *Facial ulcers*. Usually involve the alae nasi, but the cheek, forehead and malar area may also be affected. There is always a history of persistent self-inflicted trauma. Intra-oral ulceration is rare.

**Investigation of Trigeminal Sensory Loss**　(1) Exclude dental causes.
(2) A full neurological assessment and examination of the post nasal space is essential.
(3) Radiography of the base of the skull (for erosion of foramina), maxillary sinuses and jaws.
(4) Blood tests — ESR and serology.
(5) If the aetiology is not established prolonged follow-up is necessary.

**Motor**　The muscles of facial expression are supplied by the seventh cranial nerve. Facial weakness may be due to primary muscle disease (e.g. myasthenia gravis) or to nerve lesions.

**Anatomy of the Facial Nerve**　The facial nerve is a motor nerve, with a small sensory component of taste and secretory fibres. The motor nucleus lies in the pons. The pontine neurones which control movement of the upper part of the face are innervated from both cerebral hemispheres, while neurones controlling movement of the lower face are innervated only from the opposite hemisphere. Fibres cross the cerebellopontine angle after leaving the pons and enter the internal auditory meatus and facial canal. The nerve is associated in the canal with the geniculate ganglion which contains taste and secretomotor fibres. It then passes out of the stylomastoid foramen and enters the parotid gland.

**Tests of Seventh Nerve Function**

*Motor.* Lower facial muscles are tested by asking the patient to smile or 'show his teeth'. Upper facial muscles are tested by asking the patient to screw up his eyes or wrinkle the forehead.

*Taste.* This is a difficult and unsatisfactory examination. Apply sugar, salt, vinegar and quinine (sweet, salt, sour, bitter) to the tongue.

*Secretion.* Salivary secretion tests are seldom required.

**Types of Facial Weakness**

*Upper motor neurone lesion.* A lesion above the pontine nucleus causes lower facial paralysis. The upper part of the face escapes because of its bilateral innervation. Aetiology: cerebral haemorrhage, infarction and tumours.

·*Lower motor neurone lesion.* The lesion lies between the pontine nucleus and the periphery. It is characterized by paralysis of both upper and lower parts of the face. The commonest cause is Bell's palsy.

## Chapter 8  Psychiatric Disorders in Dentistry

Psychiatry has made considerable advances in recent years. This is particularly true in relation to drug treatment which has revolutionized the care of many psychiatric disorders. However, terminology and diagnosis still remain confusing, especially to the uninitiated. One reason for this is, perhaps, that psychiatry, unlike many other specialties, has the limitation of lack of scientific measurement by laboratory analysis.

There are many psychiatric problems encountered in dentistry and they have been neglected for too long. In defining dentistry one should consider the triangle of:
(1) The patient
(2) The dentist
(3) Auxillary staff
And not just consider one (e.g. the patient) in isolation.

However, the main consideration of this chapter will be on the manifestations and management of psychiatric disorders in dental patients.

**Anatomical and Physiological Considerations**

Developmental studies of oral function show that the mouth and para-oral soft tissues have the richest sensory innervation in the entire body — rivalled only by the palmer surface of the thumb. This can be proved physiologically by the two-point discrimination test. We also know that a large part of the sensory homunculus on the cerebral cortex (and therefore, a large number of brain cells) receives information from oro-facial structures.

In addition, the muscles of emotional expression and mastication function mainly in and around the mouth.

From infancy onwards the mouth is concerned intimately with the psychological development of the individual, and specific structures such as the lips, teeth, and oral mucosa (especially the tongue) can hold enormous emotional significance. The major instincts for survival of the individual are expressed in food intake and hostility or aggression and those concerned with survival of the species are expressed in sexual behaviour.

Finally, in diagnosis, one should try to determine which came first:

(1) The mental disorder which resulted in the oral manifestation, or
(2) The oral disorder, such as chronic pain, which gave rise to the mental disorder.

**Clinical Considerations**
Oral aspects of psychiatry can involve every clinical specialty of dentistry and the patient's age can range from childhood to old age. General dental practice today is a highly complex procedure and in some ways one could say that the more successful the practitioner, the better a 'psychiatrist' he is. He or she is concerned not only with pain control; treatment may interfere with many other aspects of the patient's emotional make-up. The importance of this fact is compounded by the ever increasing number of litigation cases against the profession.

**Classification**
Classification can be highly complex. A simple approach which enables one to determine management and referral is:
(1) Neurosis — insight present
(2) Psychosis — insight absent
(3) Psychosomatic disorders
(4) Mental retardation
There are, of course, many subdivisions in each group.

**Neurosis**
A neurotic illness is associated with mood changes, usually anxiety or depression, the essential feature of which is that the patient has insight; he or she is aware of the illness and may even ask 'could it be due to my nerves?'. A neurosis most frequently presents as an anxiety state or a depression.

*Anxiety*
The diagnosis of anxiety can be made by a relevant history together with systemic manifestations of over activity of the sympathetic system. Every system potentially can be affected especially in acute anxiety — common findings are elevated blood pressure and rapid pulse (which returns to normal during sleep), increased respiration, increased muscle tone, especially in the muscles of mastication and brisk reflexes, dilated pupils, hand and tongue tremor, perspiration, indigestion and intestinal hurry, restlessness and insomnia. These physical changes probably result from increased activity of the adrenal medulla and cortex which result in higher levels of catecholamines and corticosteroids in the blood. The thyroid gland may also play a part in the resultant increased metabolism.

Temporomandibular joint dysfunction may be associated with anxiety.

*Depression*

Depression may be a complication of untreated anxiety, it may follow mental trauma, or it may arise spontaneously. The clinical picture will probably be in sharp contrast to anxiety with a reduction in activity in different systems. This is an important consideration in management because therapy with a benzodiazepine such as diazepam alone may make the depression worse. Specific anti-depressive agents should be used.

Chronic facial pain, sore tongue and dry mouth are some of the common findings in depression.

*Other neuroses*

Obsessional, phobic, hysterical and hypochondrical neuroses are recognized and are generally more resistant to treatment.

**Psychoses**

In a psychotic illness insight, or contact with reality, may be reduced or lost altogether. Psychoses form the major group of psychiatric illnesses, and three main types — affective (or anxiety/depressive) psychosis, schizophrenia, and paranoia are recognized.

Facial pain, inability to wear dentures and occasionally bizarre complaints may be associated with psychoses but the patient will refuse to recognize a mental or emotional factor in spite of reassurance and extensive investigations.

The dental management of psychotic patients can be very difficult for everyone concerned and many litigation cases have resulted. The dental practitioner should try to recognize psychotic illness as early as possible so that he can take steps to avoid such an outcome.

**Psychosomatic Disorders**

Psychosomatic disorders are actual physical diseases which may be produced or aggravated by emotional disturbances. There are many examples in other parts of the body and include peptic ulceration, hypertension, asthma and eczema.

Any structure in and around the mouth may show evidence of a psychosomatic disorder. The following classification may help:

1. *Teeth.* Bruxism can lead to obvious changes in enamel, dentine, pulp and periodontal structures including the supporting bone. Nail biting may also be present.

2. *Oral mucosa.* Lips and cheek biting are common

minor psychosomatic disorders. Stomatitis artefacta is a more serious oral manifestation. It occurs in the form of deliberate self-inflicted injury often repeated in the same area with a sharp instrument.
Aphthous ulceration, lichen planus, erythema multiforme, benign migratory glossitis (geographic) are often labelled psychosomatic. Pemphigoid, herpes labialis and Vincent's infection may be associated with emotional problems.
Leukoplakia resulting from smoking or from the application of other mucosal irritants as in submucous fibrosis are examples of lesions produced by neurotic habits.
Symptoms arising from the oral mucosa such as sore tongue, altered taste or a generalized 'burning mouth' in the absence of clinical signs are further examples. One should always consider the possibility of a cancerphobia in these cases.
3. *Temporomandibular joints.* Pain arising in and around these joints can sometimes be psychosomatic.
4. *Salivary glands.* Xerostomia and, more rarely, ptyalism may result from emotional disturbances.

**Mental Retardation**

This implies a state of arrested mental development and the clinical picture can vary greatly. Patients may develop oral disease through lack of care. In addition, the tongue may be enlarged in cretinism and mongolism.
In spite of the mental handicap these patients require dental treatment similar to normal people. In this way their oral disease can be reduced to a minimum.

**Psychogenic Pain**

Pain is probably the commonest psychiatric problem in dentistry and may be associated with many emotional disorders.
If the patient continues to complain in the absence of clinical and laboratory findings then a psychological disturbance should be considered.
The common forms of psychogenic pain are detailed below.

*Glossopyrosis*

Although the tongue is most frequently involved the patient may also complain of burning lips and gums which may interfere with the ability to wear dentures.
Examination will be negative but patients will persist and may say that 'the burning sensation is getting worse'. It is usually bilateral and often relieved by eating and drinking in contrast to inflammatory lesions which are made worse by food.

Laboratory screening for anaemia and candidal infection may be undertaken. A cancerphobia is frequently associated with a glossopyrosis.

*Atypical facial pain*

Atypical facial pain is a relatively common condition and seems to occur more frequently in middle-aged women. The pain is usually a dull continuous ache more often affecting the upper jaw. It may be bilateral and can have a large area of reference. There is a poor response to analgesics and the effect of a local anaesthetic injection, or ointment applied topically, will probably be minimal. In some cases it can make the pain worse. Several unsuccessful oral surgical procedures may have been carried out.

Many such patients are depressed. They may admit to mood alteration, irritability, emotional instability and sometimes early morning waking. The symptoms are probably more often found in atypical facial pain than the TM joint pain dysfunction.

Unfortunately, a number of these patients may lack insight and will persist in blaming peripheral organic diseases for their pain. Initially, many will turn down psychiatric help but will willingly submit to surgery if it is offered.

*Temporomandibular joint pain*

This is one of the most common causes of facial pain. Most patients are female and they tend to be younger than the atypical facial pain group.

It is generally accepted that if a person cannot express their emotions consciously to relieve tension they may be converted into somatic symptoms including pain. The mouth can express such emotions as love, hate, anger, frustration, fear and worry. The result can be reflected in abnormal function of the joint and its surrounding muscles.

Pain usually occurs on mandibular movement. There is a continuous dull ache with acute episodes. It can be referred to the temporal, mastoid and occipital regions and sometimes down the neck to the shoulders. Headache, tinnitus, chest and low back pain may also be present.

The affected joints, as well as the muscles of mastication, are usually tender. Of particular importance is the area of insertion of the temporalis muscle into the coronoid process of the mandible. Experience has shown that this is the first area for muscle tenderness to develop and the last area for it to go with TM joint pain. Deviation to the affected side and limitation of opening may also be present.

The result of joint radiographs should be unremarkable

**Management of Psychiatric Problems**

If oral lesions such as ulcers, blisters and white lesions are present then local or systemic therapy is indicated. Lichen planus, leukoplakia and aphthous ulceration are particularly important here. Also, if anaemia and nutritional deficiencies are found they should be treated.

In the absence of oro-facial lesions and laboratory findings a primary emotional cause for the complaint will have to be considered. A psychiatrist may not be necessary in the management of most mild neurotic illnesses. Anxiety can be treated by a benzodiazepine or other anxiolytic agent together with psychotherapy. Depression, associated with glossopyrosis or atypical facial pain may respond to an antidepressant such as dothiepin (Prothiaden) and counselling.

One should always be aware of a suicide risk in depression and sedatives or tranquillizers should only be prescribed with an anti-depressant as they can, on their own, make a depression worse.

Finally, there is a great need for a better understanding and more research into the many complex psychiatric problems in dentistry. It is an enormous field which appears to have been largely neglected up to now.

# Chapter 9  Medical Disorders in Dental Practice

**Rheumatic Fever**    A connective tissue disorder which may cause permanent heart damage. A patient with a suggestive history should be regarded as having permanent heart damage (regardless of ausculatory findings) unless denied by a reliable authority.

*Aetiology*    The disease is caused by beta-haemolytic streptococcus Lancefield group A (*Strep. pyogenes*). The antibody provoked by this bacterium cross-reacts specifically with cardiac tissue. Beta-haemolytic streptococcus is consistently and invariably sensitive to penicillin. Control of the disease has been achieved by long term use of penicillin.

*Heart valve lesions*    Over 50 per cent of infected children develop permanent valve lesions, of which mitral stenosis is the most common.

**Infective Endocarditis**    Infective endocarditis is an uncommon disease. Many of the classical symptoms (e.g. emboli) are due to a deposition of circulating immune complexes arising from bacterial antigen and host antibody.

*Aetiology*    Causes are: alpha haemolytic streptococcus (*Strep. viridans*) 60 per cent; staphylococcus 25 per cent; *Candida, Haemophilus, Rickettsia* and culture-negative cases 15 per cent.

*Predisposing factors*    30 per cent of patients have no underlying cardiac abnormality, although some have degenerative heart disease. Rheumatic fever 20 per cent, prosthetic valves and cardiac surgery 20 per cent (increasing importance). Malignancy, urogenital surgery, long standing i.v. infusions, narcotic abuse.

*Age*    Rare in childhood. Peak incidence of streptococcal endocarditis after fifth decade. Staphylococcal endocarditis occurs at all ages (due to narcotic abuse or cardiac surgery).

*Cardiac lesions*    Lesions with most risk are those where a high velocity jet of blood forms a vortex and damages the endocardium. Low risk lesions are those where a high velocity jet of blood cannot develop.

|                        |                        |
| ---------------------- | ---------------------- |
| *High Risk*            | *Low Risk*             |
| *Mitral incompetence*  | *Mitral stenosis*      |
| *Ventricular septal defect* | *Atrial septal defect* |
| *Aortic stenosis*      |                        |
| *Patent ductus arteriosus* |                    |
| *Any degree of mitral* |                        |
| *incompetence is significant* |                 |

**Dental Implications**

Proper prophylaxis (see below) will prevent about 10 per cent of cases of infective endocarditis.
1. Prophylaxis is required in patients with a history of:
a) Rheumatic fever or Sydenham's chorea.
b) Congenital heart disease.
c) Cardiac valve surgery.
d) Haemodialysis.
e) Previous endocarditis.
f) Arterial or bypass surgery in the previous 6 months.
2. Avoid excessive trauma and complete all extractions at one visit.
3. After one attack of endocarditis all remaining teeth should be extracted unless the oral health is excellent.
4. Prophylactic cover is required for periodontal procedures (unless minor) and endodontics. Not usually necessary for conservative treatment.

**Antibiotic Prophylaxis**

It is esential to use a bactericidal antibiotic; penicillin is the drug of choice. Regimens vary between authorities. All agree that patients with cardiac prostheses require additional antibiotics as well as penicillin. Exact rules are hard to formulate and clinical judgement must err on the side of safety.
*Dose:* Adults (over 12 years):
a) 1 megaunit of crystalline penicillin intramuscularly 30 minutes prior to surgery followed by amoxycillin 250 mg tds for 3 days.
or:
b) Amoxycillin 3 g orally given 45 minutes prior to surgery followed by 3 g, 12 hours later. (N.B. This oral dose is sufficient to produce anaphylaxis in allergic patients). Children (under 12 years) use half the adult dose.
If penicillin prophylaxis is commenced the day before treatment, resistant strains of *Streptococcus viridans* will appear in the mouth within 24 hours. To be effective, penicillin must be given 30 – 45 minutes before surgery. Patients on long term penicillin for any reason must be given an alternative antibiotic — usually erythromycin — for the same reason.

In cases of hypersensitivity to penicillin, give —
a) Cephazolin 1 g intramuscularly given 30 minutes prior to treatment followed by oral erythromycin 250 mg every 6 hours for 3 days.
or
b) Erythromycin 2 g oral given 45 minutes prior to treatment followed by 250 mg every 6 hours for 3 days. Children: half the above doses.

*Patients with Prosthetic valves*

1 megaunit of benzyl penicillin plus gentomycin 80 mg intramuscularly or streptomycin 1 g intramuscularly, followed by oral antibiotics.

**Cross Sensitivity between Penicillin and Cephalosporins**

10 per cent of patients who are allergic to penicillin are also allergic to cephalosporins. If the patient only exhibits a rash with penicillin and does not suffer from hay fever, asthma or multiple skin allergies, it is safe to prescribe a cephalosporin. Alternatively, cross-sensitivity can be checked by prescribing increasing oral doses of cephalexin at 2 hour intervals as follows — 50 mg, 100 mg, 250 mg, 500 mg, 1 g. The first two doses are given as suspension and the last 3 as capsules. If there is no reaction after 1 g, another cephalosporin can be given safely by iv or im route.

*Hip replacement*

Late infections in total joint replacement may follow transient bacteraemia. Circumstantial evidence suggests that some may arise following dental manipulations but the incidence is low. Prophylaxis is optional.

**Bleeding Disorders**

May be produced by defects in vessel walls, platelets or coagulation mechanism.

*Investigation of suspected disorder*

*History:*
Previous heavy bleeding following extraction may be significant. Severe bruising and spontaneous epistaxis should not be ignored.

*Investigations*

| Test | Purpose |
|---|---|
| Bleeding and clotting time | *Not* sufficiently sensitive to be used as screening test. |
| 1. Haemoglobin | Degree of anaemia |
| 2. Platelet count | Platelet deficiency |
| 3. Prothrombin time | Plasma prothrombin level; liver disease; defects in coagulation factors. |
| 4. Thromboplastin generation time | Defects in coagulation factors. |
| 5. Capillary fragility test (Hess test) | Defects in capillary wall. |

**Anticoagulants**     Used (occasionally) in patients with prosthetic valves
or recent myocardial infarct.
There are two groups of patients on anticoagulant
therapy.
1. *Heparin group.* This is given intravenously for rapid
anticoagulation. It is used during renal dialysis.
2. *Coumarin group* (warfarin). This is given for oral
maintenance therapy. Act by interfering with
prothrombin formation and the activity of clotting
factors. It takes 24 hours to become effective and its
action can be reversed with vitamin K. Dental patients
taking anticoagulants are almost invariably in the
coumarin group.
Interactions between the coumarin drugs and other
drugs are common. In particular, salicylates, broad
spectrum antibiotics and tranquillizers inactivate the
anticoagulant. Serious bleeding may occur when
patients are taken off these groups of drugs.
Salicylates should be avoided at all times as they may
cause gastric haemorrhage and also interfere with
platelet aggregation. Unfortunately paracetamol is not
an ideal substitute, as it has a potentiating effect on
coumarin drugs.

*Management*     Patients with effective anticoagulation therapy have
prothrombin time of 21 – 36 seconds, i.e. a
prothrombin ratio 1.8 to 3.0 (control 11 – 13 seconds).
1. If a patient has regular checks on prothrombin time
and is well controlled, it is unlikely that excessive
bleeding will occur after extractions.
2. If multiple extractions are undertaken or control is
unstable, reduce the dose of anticoagulant on the day
before surgery.
3. Pay strict attention to local haemostasis.
4. Resume normal anticoagulant dose immediately
surgery is completed (the drugs take 24 hours to
become fully effective).
5. Avoid salicylates, broad spectrum antibiotics and
metronidazole.

**Cardiovascular Disease**     1. *Hypertension*
Do not alter the patient's drug therapy during
treatment, whether using local anaesthetic or general
anaesthetic. Sudden withdrawal of specific antihyper-
tensives may cause either a sudden rise or severe fall in
blood pressure. Sudden withdrawal of beta-blockaders
may precipitate angina, arrhythmia or infarction.
2. *Previous myocardial infarction*
Dental treatment and surgical procedures are stressful

and may induce angina, dysrhythmia or further infarction.
a) Avoid hypotensive episodes (pain and fear are potent hypotensives).
b) Use local anaesthesia if possible; prilocain with felypressin is the drug of choice.
c) Beta adrenergic blockade is beneficial in reducing stress. A single oral dose of atenolol 100 mg one hours before treatment is recommended if the patient is not already on beta blocking agents. Contraindications include asthma, cardiac failure and bradycardia.
d) If general anaesthesia is required, the patient should be anaesthetized in the supine position.
3. *Patients with pacemakers*
Electric currents may disrupt pacemaker function and can lead to ventricular fibrillation. Avoid using electrical equipment where possible, e.g. electric pulp testers, electrode sensitizers, electro-cautery, electro-surgery or diathermy, hyfrecator.

**Liver Disease**

Jaundiced patients should not undergo surgery.
1. Jaundice due to obstruction is associated with low prothrombin levels and patients have a bleeding tendency. This is reversed by intra-muscular vitamin K.
Alcoholics have grossly disturbed liver function and may bleed due to low prothrombin.
2. Halothane-induced jaundice following general anaesthesia is rare. It appears to be due to an abnormal metabolic process in the breakdown of halothane in the liver. Subsequent exposure to halothane carries a high mortality. Many previously reported cases are now known to have Gilbert's disease of the liver.

*Hepatitis*

Viral hepatitis is separated into 3 diseases, clinically similar but with different aetiologies.
1. *Hepatitis A.* caused by hepatitis A virus (HAV), known previously as infectious hepatitis. It is common, endemic and not transmitted by blood transfusion. It is spread by the faecal – oral route and carrier states do not occur. It can be identified by specific antibody tests.
2. *Hepatitis B.* (serum hepatitis) is caused by hepatitis B virus (HBV). It may cause serious liver disease and occasionally death. The dentist is at risk if he has treated infected patients, and can transmit the disease to other people. It is blood-borne and associated with carrier states.

**3. *Non A- Non B- hepatitis.*** This involves more than one virus and the diagnosis is made by excluding HAV and HBV. No specific antibody tests are available for identification. It is the major cause of transfusion hepatitis. It is blood-borne and carrier states exist.

*Hepatitis B*  Certain groups of people have an increased incidence of hepatitis B. They include drug addicts, institutionalized patients (prisons and long-stay hospitals) renal dialysis patients, multiple blood transfusion patients (haemophiliacs) tatooed patients, male homosexuals and those with a recent history of jaundice.

*Serology*

The surface antigen (HB$^s$Ag, previously called Australian antigen) is part of the outer shell of the virus. It appears in the incubation period and persists into the acute phase, usually disappearing before convalescence. In a small group of people the antigen does not clear and these are referred to as chronic carriers. Antibody to surface antigen appears in convalescence. The 'e' antigen — (HB$^e$Ag) is part of the core of the virus and is associated with high infectivity. Antibody to core (anti HB$^e$) develops during the acute phase and persists after recovery. When present it indicates that the patient is not infective.

*Significance*

The presence of HB$^s$Ag does not prove that the entire virus is in the blood, but for practical purposes it is considered as the indicator of infectivity.

Any patient with surface antibody is considered to be immune to further infection. A better indication is given by the HB$^e$Ag/anti HB$^e$ system, which is not measured routinely.

*Transmission*

HBV is transmitted most efficiently by blood but saliva, tears, sweat and semen also implicated.

*Management*

All patients at risk should be tested for surface antigen prior to treatment. If they are negative, there is no risk. If positive, do not treat except in emergency. Wear gown, face mask, gloves and goggles. Avoid venepuncture. Do not use the air turbine (although risk from aerosol spread is small). The patient spits into a closed plastic bag; use disposable equipment and clothing which can be incinerated. Items such as pens, pencils, dental records or the telephone should not be touched by hands or gloves contaminated with blood or saliva.

Prosthetic appliances and impressions should be washed and placed in a 2 per cent solution of glutaraldehyde before sending to the laboratory. Instruments should be washed and autoclaved and those which cannot be sterilized by heat should be soaked in 2 per cent glutaraldehyde for 1 hour. Carrier status patients can be treated for routine dentistry but the above precautions must be taken. These patients are considered infective unless anti-HB$^e$ can be demonstrated.

*Accidental innoculation*  Definite exposure occurs when blood or saliva from an HB$^S$Ag patient comes in contact with a cut in the skin, or the intact mucosa of the mouth or conjunctiva. The surgeon should be tested immediately for Hb$^S$Ab and if this is present, no further action need be taken. If there is no Hb$^S$Ab present, 4 ml of human hepatitis B immunoglobulin must be given intramuscularly and repeated 4 weeks later.

**Anti-Depressants**  1. *Monoamine oxidase inhibitors (MAOIs)*
Dangerous interactions with some drugs have been recorded, e.g. pethidine, atrophine and barbiturates. Great caution must be exercised if a general anaesthetic is given.
Although the enzyme monoamine oxidase plays some part in the breakdown of adrenaline and nor-adrenaline at nerve endings, the enzyme catechol-*o*-methyltransferase is predominantly responsible. Therefore, local anaesthetics containing adrenaline and nor-adrenaline are not contraindicated — but for absolute safety prilocaine with felypressin is the drug of choice.
2. *Tricyclic and tetracyclic antidepressants*
Significant interaction occur between these drugs and adrenaline and nor-adrenaline and local anaesthetics with these vasoconstrictors should not be used. Prilocaine with felypressin may be used safely. There are no specific contra-indications to general anaesthesia. A small number of children are prescribed tricyclic drugs for the treatment of bed wetting.
3. Patients on anti-depressants are often on combinations of several drugs. Under general anaesthesia, interactions may lead to hypotension or delayed recovery.

**Sickle Cell Disease**  Sickle cell haemoglobin (HbS) is inherited as a homozygous or heterozygous condition. It affects Africans (25%), West Indians (10%), Greeks and

Italians. Under certain conditions the erythrocytes alter shape and are unable to function properly. This may produce a venous thrombosis.

*Factors predisposing to sickling*

1. *Anoxia.* General anaesthesia is a factor of great importance. So also is flying at high altitudes.
2. *Infection.* Dental sepsis may precipitate an emergency.
3. *Cold.* Also dehydration and acidosis.

*Management*

1. All patients considered to be at risk must be screened for abnormal haemoglobins.
2. Where possible treat patients with local anaesthetic using drugs with reduced vasoconstrictor content.
3. If a general anaesthetic is required, anoxia must be scrupulously avoided.

**Corticosteroid Therapy**

Exogenous systemic corticosteroids suppress adrenal function. This may occur for up to 2 years following therapy and will inhibit normal cortisone output in 'stress' situations. Patients who are on corticosteroids or who have received treatment within the past 2 years for more than 2 weeks require adrenal supplements for surgery.

*Local anaesthetics*

Out-patient basis; cases of simple extractions and other minor procedures. Give double the usual oral daily corticosteroid dose 6 hours before operation or give 100 mg i.m. hydrocortisone sodium succinate half hour before operation. Recommence normal oral dose the same day.

*Hospital admission*

| *Patients currently on corticosteroids —* | *Patients previously on corticosteroids —* |
|---|---|
| Day of operation: | Day of operation: |
| Normal oral dose prior to fasting. Hydrocortisone 100 mg i.m. with premed, and repeat 6 hourly for 24 hours | 100 mg i.m. hydrocortisone succinate with premed, repeat 6 hour post op. Monitor blood pressure. |
| Recommence oral dose as soon as possible. | No further steroids unless blood pressure falls. |

N.B. Infection increases cortisone requirements.

**Diabetes Mellitus**

Two groups of patients:
Juvenile onset (under 40). These patients require insulin.
Mature age onset. These patients are usually controlled by diet, alone or with drugs.

*Complications of dental significance*  1. *Infection.* Diabetics are prone to infection. Minor infections in patients on insulin must be regarded as serious.
2. *Atherosclerosis.* Develops commonly and in a younger age group than normal. Remember that insidious myocardial disease may be present.
3. *Hypoglycaemia.* Usually a problem associated with patients on insulin but may occur with other hypoglycaemic agents. The brain can only store limited amounts of carbohydrate, and therefore is sensitive to severe or recurrent hypoglycaemia which leads to permanent damage. General anaesthesia should be avoided in unstabilized or severely infected patients.

*Management*  Antibiotics should be given preoperatively.

*Local anaesthetic cases*  No special preoperative measures are necessary apart from antibiotic protection.

*General anaesthetic cases*  Most patients are able to eat within 24 hours.
*Dietary controlled patients:* Preoperative starvation only.
*Oral drug controlled patients:* Omit drugs when preoperative fasting commences and resume normal dose when the patient can eat.
*Insulin patients:* Regimen varies considerably between anaesthetists.
If the patient will be able to eat within 24 hours do not change a long acting preparation to soluble insulin. Give normal diet and normal dose of insulin and operate on the patient about 4 hours later. Give 50 ml of 50 per cent glucose intravenously during the anaesthetic if desired and recommence dietary intake as soon as possible.
If the patient cannot eat for some days change long acting insulin to soluble variety. Set up dextrose drip and monitor the urine and blood sugar level, adjusting the insulin requirements accordingly.

# Chapter 10  Saliva and Salivary Gland Disorders

Saliva is produced from the major and minor salivary glands by two types of reflexes — unconditioned and conditioned. The normal and pathological functions of saliva include:

1. *Taste*

Sweet, sour, salt and bitter modalities are recognized. A specific substance must be soluble in water before the taste mechanism is fired. In addition the secretion of saliva can reflexly initiate gastric and pancreatic secretions. It also forms a powerful protection against poisonous substances. There is a difference between taste and flavour perception; the latter is a combination of gustatory and olfactory input and has an enormous range.

2. *Lubrication*

Speech, chewing and swallowing are dependant upon adequate lubrication. In addition to the water content, salivary mucin is important in this regard.

3. *Buffer*

A buffer is a substance in solution which inhibits, or tends to inhibit, a change in pH when an acid or alkali is added. Bicarbonates, phosphorus and proteins are the main buffers in saliva.

4. *Pathological aspects*

Certain micro-organisms can be found in saliva and form the basis for droplet infection. Hepatitis, poliomyelitis, measles, mumps, influenza, herpes simplex and rabies are some infections that can be spread in this way.

Body constituents such as sugar and urea may be detectable under certain circumstances. Chemicals and drugs may be found on salivary analysis in some patients; these include thiocyanates, mercury, lead, potassium and iodine.

Blood groups can be determined from samples of salivary and this fact can be important in forensic work.

5. *Digestion*

The only digestive function of saliva is in relation to carbohydrate; salivary amylase can break down starch as far as maltose.

6. *Water balance*

Water balance of the body is maintained through

equilibration of water gained from fluids, food and oxidation of hydrogen in food and water lost through urine, skin, respiration, and faeces. In the early stages of dehydration, from whatever cause, the thirst reflex will operate and will compel the patient to replace lost fluid.

7. *Cleansing*
This refers to the mechanical function of removing debris from the teeth and oral mucosa.

8. *Coagulation of blood*
In the presence of saliva shed blood will clot more quickly. Salivary mucin seems to be important in this mechanism.

9. *Chemotaxis*
Saliva exerts positive chemotaxis in the presence of infection. Also, lyzozyme, leukotaxin, opsonins and other bacterial antagonists have been demonstrated in saliva.

10. *Immunological function*
Saliva also contains antibodies which can be important in respiratory infection.

*Changes in salivary flow*

Changes in salivary flow can be considered under:
a) Quality. Composition may vary.
b) Quantity. Changes in quantity of saliva can be caused by:
(i) Physiological factors such as anxiety, sleep and increasing age.
(ii) Pathological factors; the results may be xerostomia or ptyalism.

**Xerostomia**

This can be classified as true or false.
*True xerostomia*
1. *Developmental causes.* Aplasia or hypoplasia of glandular tissue and atresia of ducts may cause selective true xerostomia.
2. *Trauma.* Mechanical or surgical removal of salivary glands, damage to nerve pathways and sialolithiasis.
3. *Inflammatory causes* — local
(i) *Infections:* Acute parotitis, mumps, uveoparotid fever, TB and sarcoidosis. (ii) *Non-infection:* Sicca syndrome, Sjörgen's syndrome, Mikulicz's syndrome, Mikulicz's disease.
These are referred to later under salivary gland disease.
— General: acute febrile conditions.
4. *Drugs.* Atropine, antihistamines, zinc poisoning, probanthine, ephedrine, aldomet, tricyclic and tetracyclic antidepressants.

5. *Metabolic causes.* Dehydration, shock, diabetes, haemorrhage, cardiac and renal failure, menopause, senility and toxic goitre.
6. *Neoplastic causes.* Benign or malignant salivary tumours.
7. *Nutritional causes.* Vitamin A deficiency, anaemia (iron).
8. *Radiation-induced.*
9. *Psychiatric causes.* Neurosis and psychosis.

B. *False*
1. Mouth breathing
2. Auriculo-temporal syndrome
3. Psychiatric

**Ptyalism**

Ptyalism can be classified as true or false.
*True ptyalism.* Causes are
(i) *Stimulation of the afferent are*
a) Mouth — full dentures, teething, foreign bodies, infections.
b) Reflex — Oesophagus, stomach, pregnancy.
c) Specific Fevers, e.g. rabies, smallpox.
(ii) *Salivary gland damage*
d) Drugs, e.g. pilocarpine, heavy metals.
e) Infections, e.g. syphilis.
f) Vitamin deficiency, e.g. pellagra.
(iii) *CNS lesions*
g) Bulbar lesions.
h) Meniere's disease and GPI.
i) Psychoses, hysteria

*False ptyalism. Causes:*
a) Facial paralysis
b) Tongue lesions
c) Oesophagus
d) Cardiospasm
e) Psychiatric

**Salivary Gland Disease**

Disease may affect either major or minor glands. The parotid is involved more frequently than the other glands.

*Acute swellings*

Viral Parotitis. Myxovirus (mumps) occurs mainly in children. Coxsackie group A viruses, lymphocytic-choriomeningitis and Echovirus infections are rare. Bacterial parotitis often follows surgery but is uncommon since the advent of antibiotics.

*Chronic recurrent swellings*

Most commonly due to obstruction (from calculi) or the sicca (dry) syndrome. Infection may be superimposed on any disorder associated with reduced salivary flow. This produces further obstruction often making the primary diagnosis difficult.

**Calculi**  Stated to be three times more common in the submandibular than the parotid gland, but the smaller duct of the latter may be occluded by calculi which are difficult to demonstrate.

*Clinical features*  May be asymptomatic or present with pain and recurrent glandular swelling which in the early stages is related to meals. In the later stages infection is super-imposed and the relationship to meals becomes less obvious, particularly in the parotid. Dryness of the mouth is not a feature.

*Investigations*  Radiographs: plain films reveal a radiopaque calculus in many cases.
Sialogram: 'large duct sialectasis' is found in well established cases. Dilation of the main ducts distal to the obstruction and branch duct changes occur.
Secretion studies: reduced secretion is found on the affected side.
Curry's Test: a means of demonstrating the rate of parotid secretion. 5 mg of pilocarpine is injected intravenously and the saliva collected from each parotid gland over a five minute period. The normal range is 3 to 13 ml. The test is most valuable in demonstrating unilateral disease.

**Sicca Syndrome**  Also known as 'benign lympho-epithelial lesion of the parotid,' but it affects all the major and minor glands around the mouth and eyes.

*Aetiology*  Probably an autoimmune disorder in which the secretory salivary lobules are replaced with lymphoid tissue.

*Sex and age*  Most common in women; occurs in middle age.

*Clinical features*  Recurrent swelling of the salivary or lacrymal glands which may be unilateral. Dryness of the mouth occurs and eventually there is a total absence of all secretion.

*Investigations*  *Sialogram:* 'Punctuate sialectasis' is seen in the early stages. No dilation of large ducts occur but the radiopaque material penetrates the substance of the gland at the intralobular level. This appearance has not been described in the submandibular gland.
*Secretion studies:* Reduced secretion occurs bilaterally.
*Blood:* The ESR is raised. Rheumatoid factor, antinuclear factor, thyroid antibodies and gastric antibodies have been demonstrated in many patients.

*Lip biopsy:* Shows: 1. Accumulation of lymphocytes around duct walls. 2. Replacement of salivary lobules with lymphoid tissue. 3. Dilated and fibrosed ducts.

**Sjörgen's Syndrome** A triad consisting of:
1. Kerato-conjunctivitis sicca.
2. Xerostomia.
3. Connective tissue disorders (including rheumatic arthritis).
Glandular enlargement may not occur.
The condition is similar to the sicca syndrome but with the emphasis on its generalised nature.

**Mikulicz's Disease** Mikulicz originally described a patient with progressive enlargement of the lacrymal submandibular and (finally) the parotid gland. His histological findings on the lacrymal gland suggest that the patient was suffering from the sicca syndrome.

**Mikulicz's Syndrome** A term used in the past to describe any enlargement of the parotid gland. It should be discarded and lesions classified according to the aetiology of the swelling, e.g. sarcoidosis, amyloidosis and leukaemia.

**Other Causes of Parotid Swelling**
1. *Obstruction*
(i) Stricture.
(ii) Trauma to parotid papilla, e.g. denture flange.
(iii) Impaction of a foreign body.
2. *Metabolic*
(i) Cirrhosis of liver.
(ii) Diabetes and disturbed glucose metabolism.
3. *Drugs*
Phenylbutazone, thiouracil and phenothiazines.
4. *Pneumo-parotitis*
Glass blowing, wind instrument blowing and surgical emphysema.
5. *Work hypertrophy*
Starch ingestion.
6. *Chronic granulomatous conditions*
Sarcoid (6% of all sarcoid cases involve the parotid).

**Neoplastic Disease** Major glands are affected ten times more often than minor glands, and parotid glands are affected ten times more often than than submandibular glands.
Single lumps arising in the salivary glands are very difficult to diagnose clinically. The correct treatment of parotid lumps is resection with a margin of surrounding healthy salivary tissue. In the

submandibular it is easier to remove the entire gland

**Major Gland Neoplasms — non-Malignant**

*Pleomorphic adenoma* (mixed parotid tumour): 80 per cent of all cases are non-malignant. Usually found in parotid during 3rd to 4th decade. Equal sex distribution. Slow growing circumscribed and seldom involves facial nerve.

*Adenolymphoma.* (Warthin's tumour or papillary cystadenoma lymphomastosum). Rare outside parotid; 90 per cent of patients males in 5th to 6th decade. Slow growing, fluctuant, often multiple or bilateral and usually situated in the lower pole.

*Adenoma* (rare).

*Oxyphil cell adenoma* (rare).

**Malignant**

*Pleomorphic adenoma.* 60 per cent of malignant tumours. Long standing benign lesions may suddenly become aggressive, or the tumour may only have a short history. Facial paralysis or ulceration is a sinister omen.

Adenocystic carcinoma (15%), (cylindroma or basiloma). Growth associated with pain and ulceration and spreads via the perineural lymphatics.

Adenocarcinoma (10%).

Mucoepidermoid carcinoma (10%).

Squamous cell carcinoma (5%).

Acinar cell carcinoma (rare).

**Minor Gland Tumours**

The palate is the most frequent site for all minor gland tumours. Other sites are the upper lip (pleomorphic adenoma), the tongue and retromolar area. A high percentage in the retromolar region are malignant.

*Approximate incidence*

Pleomorphic adenoma 55 per cent (70 per cent of them are benign).

Adenocystic carcinoma (malignant) 15 – 25 per cent.

Mucoepidermoid carcinoma (malignant) 25 – 30 per cent.

Adenocarcinoma (malignant) 5 per cent.

Squamous cell carcinoma less than 1 per cent.

*Mesenchymal tumours*

Fibroma, lipoma, haemangioma, neurofibroma and their malignant counterparts are rare in salivary glands.

*Minor gland disease*

A mucocoele is often found on the lower lip but may occur at any site where minor glands exist. Two varieties are recognised.

(i) Mucous extravasation 'cyst'. Following trauma to

the duct of a minor gland, mucus is released into the tissues and is surrounded by fibrous or granulation tissue without epithelium lining the wall of the cyst.
(ii) Mucus retention cyst. A less common variety. Trauma results in partial obstruction of the mucous glands; duct dilation and epithelial proliferation results in a cavity lined with epithelium.
*Ranula.* This is the clinical diagnosis for any lump in the floor of the mouth. In most cases it is a mucocoele involving the sublingual glands and this may be of the extravasation or retention variety.

| | |
|---|---|
| *Clinical features* | Pink translucent sac on the floor of the mouth. Fluctuant and contains mucus. May extend into the neck or base of skull (burrowing ranula). |
| *Sialolithiasis* | Calcification of the gland. |

## Chapter 11 Disorders of the Tongue and Abnormalities of Taste

The dorsal surface of the tongue is covered with thick keratinized stratified squamous epithelium forming the filiform, fungiform and circumvallate papillae which bear taste buds. The epithelium has a rapid turnover which decreases with age.

Adequate mineral and vitamin supplies are essential for cell enzyme systems and latent deficiencies may be reflected in the tongue surface. Aggregations of lymphoid tissue (lingual tonsil) occur in the posterior region on the dorso-lateral surfaces and may become inflamed and sore — a common cause of cancerphobia. The ventral surface is lined by thin non-keratinized epithelium with a few minor salivary glands.

**Developmental Lesions**

1. *Migratory glossitis* (Geographic tongue). About 10 per cent of the population are affected. Commonly females over 40 but even children suffer. Occurs as multiple red patches on the dorsal and lateral surfaces (but ventral surface can be involved) spreading across the surfaces in periods from a few days to months. Biopsy reveals an inflammatory reaction in the underlying tissue, but the lesions are harmless. No treatment is indicated.

2. *Lingual thyroid.* A rare lesion found in children on the posterior dorsal surface in the region of the foramen caecum. Presents as a lump of varying size and may produce dysphagia, dysphonia, dyspnoea or hoarseness, but most cases are asymptomatic. It may be the only functioning thyroid tissue in the body or the patient may be euthyroid.
*Treatment:* If active, suppress with antithyroid agents or surgery if size increased with age.

3. *Granular cell myoblastoma* (Abrikosov's tumour) is a benign hamartoma occurring in adults and children. About one third occur on the tongue (lateral surface usually) and the remainder elsewhere in the mouth. It is a small solitary nodule of uncertain aetiology — perhaps myogenous, neural or histiocytic. Diagnosis by excision biopsy.

4. *Median rhomboid glossitis* (Central papillary atrophy of tongue). Traditionally considered to arise from persistent tuberculum impar but some cases may

be chronic hyperplastic candidiasis. Occurs in the middle third on the tongue as smooth (absent papillae) reddened and sometimes elevated lesion 0.5 to 2.0 cm in size. Uncommon in children and occasionally irritative, neoplastic change is very rare. True aetiology may be persistent tuberculum impar which is more susceptible to invasion by candida. Uncomfortable lesions respond to antifungal therapy.

5. *Angio-oedema.* May be hereditary or non-hereditary. Caused by a marked reduction of the inhibitor of the first component of complement (C$^1$ esterase inhibitor) affecting the fibrinolytic, kinin-generating and complement systems. The hereditary variety shows a strong family history (autosomal dominant) but may present at any time from childhood to old age for the first time. The symptoms include brawny non-pitting oedema of the face (including tongue) and extremities, and abdominal pain. Urticaria and rashes are absent and there is no history of allergy.

The non-hereditary variety is similar except the patients are always adults and there is no family history.

Dental manipulations are notorious for precipitating life-endangering swellings of the mouth and pharynx in these patients, and dental extractions should be performed in hospital after prophylaxis with fresh frozen plasma and anti-fibrinolytic drugs. Treatment of acute attacks is unsatisfactory without response to corticosteroids adrenaline or antihistamines. Emergency tracheostomy may be life saving. Long term prophylaxis with antifibrinolytic drugs is effective in some patients. The Melkersson-Rosenthal syndrome, characterized by recurrent facial swelling, episodic facial palsy and fissured tongue, is probably allergic in origin.

**Infective Lesions**   1. *Viral*
a) Herpetic stomatitis follows primary contact with herpes simplex type I virus and is the commonest viral infection of the mouth. It usually affects children and young adults and principally involves the gingiva. The dorsum of the tongue is heavily coated but vesicles, which rupture after 24 hours leaving small ulcers, do occur. The lesions disappear spontaneously after 14 days but mouth rinses with carbenoxolone will clear primary lesions in three to four days. The mode of action is not known. Very few patients develop recurrent herpes simplex of the tongue.

b) Herpes zoster may present as a localized eruption following activation of a latent virus in the sensory posterior root ganglion. The tongue may be involved with unilateral vesicular lesions. Severe pain may precede the eruptions by four to five days and make diagnosis difficult. Antibody to herpes zoster decreases after middle age and attacks increase in intensity and severity. Contrary to popular belief, there is no good evidence that zoster infections suggest hidden malignancy.

c) Herpetiform ulcers occurs as a crop of 10 – 30 tiny aphthae which coalesce and heal in seven to fourteen days. Intra-nuclear inclusion bodies suggest a viral lesion but not of the herpes simplex type. Tetracycline mouth rinses can be helpful.

d) Herpangina is caused by the Coxsachie group A virus. It is a disease of children affecting the throat and mouth and sometimes the tongue. Characteristically, it does not involve the gingiva. The condition resolves within five to seven days.

e) Focal epithelial hyperplasia is an uncommon condition affecting Eskimos, Australian Aborigines, American Indians and occasionally Caucasians. Multiple modular elevations occur throughout the mouth and over the tongue. Biopsy reveals cells filled with viral particles. The condition is not premalignant.

2. *Candidiasis*

a) Acute pseudo-membraneous lesions occur in the newborn, severely ill adults, and in asthmatics using a betamethasone (steroid) inhaler. The white curdy patches are seen on the cheeks, lips, palate and tongue and when removed leave a bleeding surface.

b) Acute atrophic candidiasis may occur when taking oral antibiotics. It causes painful reddened tongue (antibiotic tongue) with associated white areas and represents a superficial fungal infection.

c) Chronic hyperplastic candidiasis (candidal leukoplakia). Occurs as:

i) part of mucocutaneous candidiasis; or as ii) isolated lesions in the mouth.

In mucocutaneous disease, the candidiasis affects the skin and nails in early life. Malignant change in the oral lesions is rare.

When the candidal infections are confined to the mouth, onset is usually in late middle age and the tongue is frequently involved. The lesions have a strong tendency to become malignant particularly when associated with reddened areas (speckled leukoplakia). In some cases, however, the candidiasis is merely a secondary feature of a pre-existing keratosis. Cryotherapy has been shown to be effective in these cases in the short term; the long term benefits have yet to be assessed. Median rhomboid glossitis is believed by some to be chronic hyperplastic candidiasis.

**3. Syphilis**

The hallmark of syphilis is the absence of pain.

*Primary lesions:* the tongue is second only to the lip as the oral site for the chancre. Commences as a papule 9 – 90 days after an infection which erodes and becomes ulcerated. It is painless, hard and punched out; the associated cervical glands are hard and non-tender. The lesions last two to four weeks and heal without scarring. Dark-field examination in the mouth is unreliable for diagnosis as *Treponema pallidum* cannot be distinguished from other oral treponemas which occur normally in the oral cavity.

Secondary lesions follow the chancre by 9 – 90 days, frequently when the chancre is still healing. This phase may last two years, but a generalized painless lymphadenopathy is common. The mucous patch is an oval, raised shallow lesion covered by a greyish white membrane which occurs on the sides and tip of the tongue. Several may coalesce to form snail track ulcers.

Tertiary lesions occur 10 – 20 years after infection in about two thirds of untreated patients. Isolated gummas of the tongue are rare, but diffuse gummatous infiltration causes ischaemia and leads to chronic interstitial glossitis. The tongue surface is atrophic, thin and wrinkled, but deep lobulations and irregular fissures occur. Areas of hypertrophy present as leukoplakia, and these lesions are pre-cancerous.

**4. Tuberculosis**

Oral tuberculosis is rare but the tongue is most commonly affected. Presents as painful ulcers on the posterior surface secondary to lesions elsewhere in the body (usually lung). The lymph nodes are not affected. In primary tuberculosis, oral lesions are extremely uncommon. Seen in children as a single painless ulcer on the gingiva with enlarged lymph nodes.

**Nutritional glossitis**

Glossitis is a common manifestation of nutritional deficiencies.

**a) Iron**

The most common haematological deficiency. Blood examination reveals a hypochromic microcytic anaemia. As body iron stores fall, serum iron is reduced, the total iron-binding capacity of the serum is elevated, and the per cent saturation may also be reduced. The haemoglobin level may remain within the normal range in the early stages until the body iron stores are depleted; glossitis, due to iron deficiency, may present before anaemia occurs as measured by the haemoglobin level. (In anaemia due to chronic infection or malignancy, the total iron binding capacity of the serum is not altered).

*Clinical signs*   Pallor is unreliable but may occur with a low haemoglobin. Glossitis presents as redness of the tongue tip which spreads over the entire dorsal surface. It is an early sign of iron deficiency. Loss of the fungiform and filiform papillae produce a smooth surface and a patchy atrophy with thinning of the mucosa. Localized areas of hyperkeratosis probably represent a response to local irritation. As the deficiency advances, the epithelium becomes eroded leaving shallow ulcers resembling aphthae which may be preceded by vesicles. Occasionally in severe cases large chronic ulcers are seen surrounded by areas of hyperkeratosis which may resemble carcinoma.

b) *Vitamin B12*
Deficiency results in a megaloblastic macrocytic anaemia.
Glossitis may be the earliest sign. The initial sign is a tender red tip which spreads over the entire dorsum. This active inflammatory reaction produces the red raw beefy tongue which later regresses as the filiform, fungiform and circumvallate papilla atrophy. Finally the entire tongue is smooth and atrophic, prone to traumatic ulceration and surface erosion. The ventral surface may also become reddened and sore and small ulcers similar to aphthae appear. Angular cheilitis is rare in vitamin B12 deficiency.
The tongue changes are reversed rapidly following specific therapy.

c) *Folic acid*
Malabsorption syndromes are the commonest cause but also cytotoxic drugs, anticonvulsants and pregnancy will cause symptoms. The clinical signs and haematological features are similar to a lack of vitamin B12 but angular cheilitis always occurs in folic acid deficiency. Oral therapy with folic acid reverses the symptoms including those caused by malabsorption syndromes. However, it should be remembered that large and prolonged doses of folic acid can lower the blood concentration of vitamin B12 and it should

*never* be given alone in treatment of pernicious anaemia or other B12 macrocytic anaemias because of the risk of precipitating subacute combined degeneration of the spinal cord.

**Dermatological Conditions**

1. *Lichen planus*
The tongue is the second most frequently involved oral organ in lichen planus (buccal mucosa is the most common) and clinical confirmation of tongue lesions should always be looked for in the cheeks. Non-erosive lichen occurs as plaque-like lesions which may cover the entire dorsum in severe cases. There are both atrophic and hyperkeratotic areas in these plaques. Minor erosions are atrophic lesions in which the mucosa has been traumatised, but may follow the rupture of a bullae. They are slow to develop and recover. There are often hyperkeratotic areas close to the borders of the erosions. Major erosions are rare but the entire dorsal surface of the tongue, together with areas of the cheeks and vestibules may be involved. The onset is rapid and the erosions cause severe discomfort. They can be intractable and resistant to treatment.

2. *Pemphigus vulgaris*
May involve the tongue but the cheeks and throat are more common. Intraepithelial bullae quickly rupture to leave slowly healing ulcerated areas. Indirect immunofluorescence will demonstrate IgG antibodies bound to intercellular areas in the epithelium.

**Neoplasms**

The commonest malignant tumour (95 per cent) is squamous cell carcinoma. Adenocarcinoma of minor salivary glands and other primary tumours are rare but include lymphoma, malignant melanoma, fibrosarcoma, rhabdomyosarcoma and plasmacytoma. Secondary deposits may also occur.

a) *Squamous cell carcinoma.* The lateral border (65 per cent) and dorsal surface are common sites. Ventral surface is involved in 10 per cent of cases. Induration is a most important sign and clinical presentation is as red, white or ulcerated area which may be relatively painless. Affects males more frequently than females (2 : 1) and usually over 50 years with history of tobacco use. Relationship to alcohol is not straightforward. Oral sepsis and local irritants are not considered major aetiological factors. Suspicious areas should have repeated biopsies as prognosis directly related to early diagnosis and size of lesion. Metastasis occurs in 30 per cent of lesions under 2 cm and 60 per cent over 2 cm.

Treatment: Surgery for small anterior mobile lesions. Radium needles or external, radiotherapy for larger lesions and those in the posterior region.

b) *Papilloma*. This is a common benign lesion occurring at any age. It is a pedunculated white swelling which should be excised. It is not premalignant.

c) *Lymphangio-haemangioma*. This is a malformation of the blood vessels and lymphatic tissues causing macroglossia. Either tissue may predominate and the lesion has a raised, lobulated appearance or may bleed freely on trauma. Treatment is not required unless bleeding occurs regularly or size is unsightly.

d) *Adenoma, Lipoma, Neurofibroma*. These are uncommon.

**Miscellaneous**

1. *Hairy tongue*

This is an elongation of filiform papillae on the dorsal surface, usually in elderly patients. Colour varies from yellow to black and pigment possibly due to medicaments, food, tobacco and/or chromogenic bacteria. The condition is acquired and a low salivary pH is common. Zinc deficiency may be important and the condition is frequently found in patients having treatment for malignant disease. Treatment involves scraping the surface after softening the papillae with dilute acetylsalicylic acid.

2. *Amyloid*

Macroglossia occurs in 25 per cent of cases. A hyaline material is deposited in the tissue and probably represents disturbed immunoglobulin synthesis. Secondary amyloidosis follows chronic tissue breakdown, e.g. multiple myeloma, rheumatoid arthritis or suppurative infection. The tongue is commonly affected and soft, elastic rubbery enlargement noted. Primary amyloidosis occurs without obvious cause. The skeletal muscles including the tongue may be involved. Tumour amyloid may occur in the tongue as an isolated mass but is uncommon. The diagnosis is usually confirmed by gingival biopsy.

3. *Burning tongue*

The tongue usually appears normal. Most patients are female, middle aged or older, suggesting a hormonal cause. Follicle stimulating hormone level is high during the menopause and is the best indication of the end of ovulation. However, the response to oestrogen therapy is generally poor.

*Management*    1. Take a careful history to exclude diabetes, malabsorption syndrome or causes of xerostomia.
2. Remove local irritants — calculus, sharp tooth edges, irregularities in dentures.
3. Haematological tests to exclude iron, vitamin B12 and folate deficiency.
4. Short trial of antidepressant drugs for at least 3 weeks to exclude depression — the most common psychogenic cause. If found effective continue therapy for as long as is necessary.
5. Reassure and review.

**Abnormalities of Taste**    Taste is closely related to smell and most patients complaining of loss of taste actually suffer from loss of smell. All patients with generalized nasal congestion (e.g. common cold) suffer from diminution in sense of smell. Actual abnormalities of taste do exist however and, owing to the anatomical relationship between the chorda tympani nerve and the middle ear, ear disease should be considered in every patient with a taste abnormality.

*Anatomy*    Taste buds are found in the fungiform and circumvallate papillae of the tongue and seldom occur elsewhere in the mouth.
Taste from the tongue is relayed in the chorda tympani nerve without alternative pathways. There is virtually no overlap across the tongue midline. The chorda tympani carries.
a) Afferent nerve fibres from the taste buds of the tongue to the mid brain.
b) Efferent secretomotor fibres from the pons to the submandibular and sublingual glands. Fibres pass from the pons as the nervus intermedius, cross the cerebellopontine angle in intimate relationship with the facial nerve and enters the internal auditory meatus.
The chorda tympani leaves the facial nerve in the middle ear. It passes close to the malleus and the drum (where it is vulnerable to surgical injury) before leaving via the pterygotympanic fissure to join the lingual nerve.

*Measurement of taste*    Electrical measurement produces accurate information useful for scientific work. Traditional testing with *salt, sweet, sour* and *bitter* (salt, sugar, vinegar and quinine) offers crude qualitative results, suitable for clinical purposes. Testing must be performed at the tongue edges, as with increasing age the dorsum of the tongue becomes insensitive.

*Aetiology*     **1. *Ear***
Ear surgery is the commonest cause of taste loss.
Stapedectomy and mastoid operations are associated
with high incidence of chorda tympani damage. Taste
loss may occur or a 'metallic' taste develops. Recovery
is rare, although in unilateral cases the symptoms
diminish. Chronic middle ear disease rarely causes
taste abnormalities. An important exception is an
erosive cholesteatoma, a serious disorder, where taste
is usually completely absent.

**2. *Oral***
An unpleasant taste (cacogeusia or dysgeusia) rather
than absent taste is commonly associated with oral
factors. Patients often complain of an associated
halitosis.
A furred tongue from any cause (antibiotics, mouth
breathing, infection, smoking) will physically block
stimulants reaching the taste buds and mechanically
interfere with function. Periodontal disease and poor
oral hygiene are the principal dental causes. A single
isolated periodontal pocket is sufficient to cause
symptoms. Epithelial debris, dead cells or frank pus
from the mouth, nasopharynx or sinus, will produce
an unpleasant taste.
Infections from any oral lesion may alter taste
sensation, particularly if associated with bleeding.
Degenerating blood produces a salty taste, as does cyst
fluid.
Glossitis due to mineral or vitamin deficiency leads to
degeneration and atrophy of the tongue epithelium.
The surface becomes smooth and pale or reddened and
denuded of epithelium destroying taste buds.
Radiotherapy will damage taste buds.
Manipulation of the lingual nerve (excessive lingual
retraction in the removal of wisdom teeth) may cause
temporary post-operative taste loss.
With increasing age, the dorsum of the tongue
becomes insensitive and taste buds are mainly located
on the lateral surfaces. A relative ischaemia of the
tongue midline is a possible explanation.

**3. *Facial nerve lesions***
Loss of taste may preceed paralysis in lesions of the
facial nerve occurring central to the origin of the
chorda tympani, e.g. Bell's palsy, Ramsay Hunt
syndrome and acoustic neuroma.

**4. *Drugs***
Numerous drugs are reported as affecting taste. The
action is not understood. The taste buds may be affected
or there may be an indirect action on the cortical

tasting area. Common examples are imipramine, lincomycin, carbimazole, griseofulvin, clofibrate, lithium, phenidione, tetracycline and metronidazole.

5. *Miscellaneous*

Epilepsy may cause bizarre taste sensations. So also may endocrine disorders including hypothyroidism, adrenocortical insufficiency, pseudohypoparathyroidism, hypergonadism, pregnancy and the menopause.

Zinc deficiency is known to reduce taste and arbitrary treatment with this metal restores normal taste to some patients when a cause cannot be found.

Psychogenic illness may decrease acuity, particularly if the patient is being treated with lithium carbonate.

**Recommentations**

1. A full neurological examination is necessary. Evaluation of the sense of smell is important, including X-rays of the sinus to exclude nasal obstruction.

2. An ENT examination is required.

3. A list of drugs being taken by the patient must be obtained.

# Chapter 12  Cervical Lymphadenopathy

Approximately one third of the lymph nodes of the body are found in the neck. Systemic diseases may therefore first present in the cervical lymph glands.

**Aetiology**

*Local infections*
1. *Pyogenic.* Possible sources are ears, nose, throat, scalp, and teeth.
2. *Tuberculosis.* Nodes enlarge only in primary tuberculosis but may calcify and remain enlarged.
3. *Syphilis.* Primary stage — regional nodes affected but may be bilateral in the neck.

**General Infections**

1. *Infectious mononucleosis*
Several clinical patterns occur some of which do not have enlarged lymph nodes (hence the term 'glandular fever' should be avoided). The disease is caused by the Epstein-Barr virus (EBV).
Diagnosis:
i) Characteristic abnormal monocytes seen in the peripheral blood film;
ii) Monospot test. A slide agglutination test for heterophil antibody. It becomes positive in the first week and remains so for several weeks. False positives are rare.
2. *Toxoplasmosis*
About 30 per cent of the population of UK carry antibody indicating an infection at some time during life. The condition has been overdiagnosed and is an uncommon cause of lymphadenopathy. Caused by *Toxoplasma gondii*; active disease can be con-firmed by:
a) fluorescent test for IgM, and
b) haemagglutination test.
3. *Syphilis*
Secondary stage — generalised lymphadenopathy.

*Idiopathic*
1. *Sarcoidosis*
A chronic multisystem disease of unknown aetiology. It is the widespread involvement which leads to the diagnosis, as the isolated 'granuloma' may be produced by a variety of agents, e.g. helminths, beryllium, regional ileitis, etc. Bone changes (as occur in the mandible) are the hallmark of chronic sarcoidosis.

2. *Systemic lupus erythematosus*
Lymphadenopathy in 50 per cent of cases.
3. *Rheumatoid arthritis*
4. *Histiocytosis X*
5. *Cherubism*
6. *Pseudo lymphoma in Sjögren's disease*

**Neoplasms**

1. *Lymphomas* (reticulosis)
*Hodgkin's disease.* Painless enlarged lymph nodes are always present and often first noted in the neck. Divided histologically in order of favourable prognosis as lymphocyte predominal nodular sclerosis and lymphocyte depleted. The Sternberg-Reed cell must be present but diagnosis cannot be made on this feature alone.
*Other diseases.* Multiple painless lymph nodes with involvement of extralymphatic tissue at early stage. Several classifications exist but the presence (favourable prognosis) or absence (unfavourable) of a nodular pattern is useful. Diagnosis on histology and absence of Sternberg-Reed cells.
2. *Leukaemia*
*Acute leukaemia* — lymphoblastic and myeloblastic varieties.
*Chronic leukaemia* — chronic lymphatic type.
*Secondary deposits.*

*Management and investigation*

1. Exclude local infection.
2. Look for other lymph node enlargement.
3. Feel for liver and spleen.
4. Blood tests (Hb WBC ESR) Monospot test. Tuberculin test if nodes do not change in size in observations made one month apart.
5. Chest X-ray.
6. Biopsy gland. Non-specific biopsies should be repeated if diagnosis uncertain.

# Chapter 13    Disorders of Mandibular Movement

Restricted jaw movement is a relatively common clinical finding. The average distance between the incisal edges in an adult is 35 – 45 mm. This should be measured with a gauge and not in finger breadths. Limitation of movement may be due to trismus or ankylosis.

**Trismus**

Defined as inability to open the mouth due to reflex muscle spasm.

*Aetiology*

1. *Trauma*
*Surgical removal of wisdom teeth.*
*Local anaesthetic injection.*
a) Direct muscle fibre damage — trismus lasts only a few days.
b) Haematoma formation — rapid onset and persistent trismus over the following weeks. As the haematoma organizes, trismus changes to ankylosis and forcible opening of the mouth under general anaesthesia is necessary. Exercises are an important adjunct to treatment.
*Direct violence.* Fractures of mandible and middle third of face.
*Foreign bodies.*
a) Lacerations of muscles of mastication.
b) Oedema formation in the infratemporal space.
2. *Infection*
*Pericoronitis and sequela.* Submasseteric pterygomandibular infratemporal parapharnygeal space infections.
*Acute bacterial and viral infections.* Acute tonsilitis, parotid abscess, acute cervical lymphadenopathy and mumps.
*Chronic infections and infestations.* Actinomycosis, noma (gangrenous stomatitis) tertiary syphilis and trichinosis.

**Temporo-Mandibular Joint Disorders**

*Pain dysfunction syndrome*
Probably the most common condition affecting the TM-joint. Essentially due to nonco-ordination of the muscles acting around the joint causing trismus. The joint itself is not diseased.
*Aetiology*
Multifactoral: Interaction between stress,

parafunctional habits and occlusal irregularities in emotionally susceptible patients. Occasionally a simple occlusal irregularity is the sole cause, e.g. high occlusal contact; overerupted wisdom teeth causing a 'bite of convenience'. More frequently symptoms are related to periods of emotional stress. The condition may be secondary to other diseases, e.g. whiplash injuries or cervical spondylosis.

*Age and sex.* Female : Male = 3 : 1. Most patients are aged 15 – 40 years.

*Clinical features*
Pain in the ear or preauricular region, radiating to the temple, cheek or neck, worse in the morning. Clicking and locking of the jaws. Trismus is worse at the beginning of the day and the muscles of mastication are tender on palpation.
Also described: tinnitus, deviated jaw opening, occlusal keratosis in buccal mucosa and burning tongue. Nocturnal bruxism occurs frequently and is indicative of an underlying chronic anxiety state.

*Investigations*
Radiography characteristically does not reveal any abnormality. Arthrography may demonstrate a displaced meniscus — so called 'internal derangement' of the joint.

*Treatment*
Essentially conservative. Reassurance, rest, physiotherapy and removal of obvious occlusal irregularities. Mechanical: bite appliances and denture adjustments. Drugs: Sedative muscle relaxants, e.g. diazepam.

*Surgery*
Cases of locking which do not improve with conservative treatment will respond to enlargement of the joint space by a high condylar 'shave'. Otherwise avoid surgery.

*Prognosis*
Most cases recover but the condition has a well known tendency to recur, particularly at times of stress. Long standing cases may lead into a secondary true osteoarthritis of the joint.

4. *Central nervous system*
1. Tetanus — painless trismus develops early.
2. Encephalitis and meningitis.
3. Brain tumour or abscess.
4. Parkinson's disease.
5. Epilepsy.

5. *Drugs*
*Phenothiazine group*
Chlorpromazine (Largactil), trifluoperazine

(Stelazine), promazine (Sparine) may produce a 'grimacing syndrome' due to increased extrapyramidal activity on the first occasion the drug is taken. The complication is also noted with high doses of the drug. The treatment is to withdraw the drug and counteract with antiParkinsonian therapy, e.g. trihexphenidyl (Artane) or intravenous barbiturates.
*Strychnine*
*Ergotamine*
6. *Neoplasms*
*Nasopharyngeal carcinoma* (Trotter's syndrome: pain in the ear, middle ear deafness, and unilateral immobility of the soft palate).
Muscle involvement and spread to the motor branch of the trigeminal nerve produces trismus.
*Neoplasms* of the tongue and floor of the mouth.
*Tumours* of the infratemporal fossae are rare.
7. *Hysteria*
Organic causes should be excluded first.

**Ankylosis**  Defined as difficulty in opening the mouth due to changes within the joint (true ankylosis) or consolidation of the structures surrounding the joint (false ankylosis). The condition may be unilateral or bilateral. Facial deformity is produced if ankylosis occurs during the growth period. In the intra-articular variety, obliteration of the joint cavity occurs and the mandible fuses with the base of the skull.
Treatment is difficult. There is little place for conservative measures (exercises or mechanical devices) which aim at stretching the joint structure.
Surgical procedures directed at producing a pseudo-arthrosis may be successful in selected cases.

*Aetiology*  *Trauma*; direct violence.
a) Joint effusions — these respond to rest, heat and single injection of steroids.
b) Haemorrhage.
c) Intra-capsular fracture — these are underdiagnosed, and leads to late osteoarthritis.
d) Zygomatic arch fracture. Zygoma fuses wich coronoid.
e) Birth injury.

**Arthritis**  1. *Osteoarthritis*
a) Post traumatic — follows fracture to condyle, intra-capsular fracture or joint effusion.
b) Degenerative disease — a common disorder. Affects females more than males over the age of 50.

*Clinical features:* Pain localized to one joint produced by movement. Usually worse at the end of the day. Tenderness over joint on palpation. Crepitus both audible and on palpation. The articular surface becomes roughened and radiography demonstrates the presence of erosions and osteophytes.
*Treatment:* anti-arthritis drugs or high condylar 'shave' very effective.
*Prognosis:* Without treatment the condition resolves in 1 – 3 years.
2. *Rheumatoid arthritis*
In adults the TMJ is clinically involved only at an advanced stage. bilateral involvement is a characteristic feature. In juvenile rheumatoid (Still's disease) lesions of the joint appear early and are very destructive.
Both intra and extra-articular fibrous adhesions develop and occasionally bone ankylosis occurs.
3. *Psoriasis and gout* — rare
4. *Suppurative* — rare
Haematogenous or direct spread from acute pyogenic infection, staphylococci, pneumococci, gonococci and *Salmonella typhi.*

*Infection*
1. *Middle ear disease* — less common since the introduction of antibiotics.
2. *Pyaemia* — staphylococcal infections in particular produce suppurative arthritis.
3. *Osteomyelitis* — direct spread from infection in the ramus fractures or open wounds to involve the joint.

*Scar tissue*
This is an uncommon condition producing ankylosis by contraction of excess fibrous tissue.
*Causes:* Post-irradiation, post-neurosurgical procedures, submucous fibrosis, myositis ossificans and epidermolysis bullosa (dystrophica).
Treatment is very difficult. Mechanical exercises are unsatisfactory. Surgical removal of adhesions occasionally possible. In cases following neurosurgery, where temporalis muscle fibrosed, coronoidectomy is effective.

*Neoplasms*
1. Coronoid hyperplasia — this mechanically prevents jaw opening.
2. Primary and secondary neoplasms in the condyle are uncommon.

# Chapter 14    Occupational Hazards in Dentistry

Dental surgeons experiences a large number of hazards in their profession. It has been shown that in the United Kingdom the highest mortality rate is between the ages of 45 – 55 years. Although permanent injury or death is rarely directly related to occupation the practitioner should be fully aware of the risks involved in order to carry out preventative measures.
Patients should also be considered at risk because the terms of reference of dentistry should include a) the operator, b) auxillary staff, and c) the patient. The community could also be considered in the wider aspects.

## Hazards

**Chemicals and Drugs**    The reactions may be:
a) Local — contact dermatitis, e.g. trichloracetic acid, silver nitrate and phenol.
b) Systemic — direct intoxication, e.g. mercurialism. The oral findings in mercurialism may include salivation, metallic taste, gingivitis, ulceration and salivary gland enlargement. The general features can include diarrhoea, irritability, depression and renal involvement.
c) Hypersensitive, e.g. local anaesthetics, penicillin, toothpaste, and barbiturates.
d) Addiction and dependence, e.g. narcotics and nitrous oxide.

**Infections**    1. The common cold.
2. Herpes simplex.
3. Hepatitis.
4. Herpes zoster.
5. Herpangina.
6. Poliomyelitis.
7. Other conditions, e.g. tuberculosis, venereal diseases and eye infections. The basic principles of microbiology should be applied to prevent the spread of infectious diseases. These include thorough sterilization of surgical instruments, correct air ventilation, use of gloves and masks, refusal to carry out routine dental treament if the operator is at risk, vaccination and regular chest radiographs.

**Radiation**    The incidence of background radiation is increasing; diagnostic radiographs and radioactive isotopes are being used to a greater extent, and increased participation of dental personnel in general hospital practice are among the reasons why practitioners should be aware of radiation hazards.

Generally two factors are recognized; (1) electro-magnetic or gamma ($\gamma$) and (2) particle radiation, alpha ($\alpha$) and beta ($\beta$). The mode of action on tissue function is uncertain but may be through the mechanism of ionization which can produce proteolysis, inhibit enzymes, and denature nucleoproteins. In addition there may be a direct effect on the cell nucleus.

The effects of radiation will depend on:
1. The amount.
2. Source — whether gamma or particle.
3. Types of filtration used.
4. Area of tissue irradiated.
5. Total time of exposure.

*Information sources*    Our knowledge of radiation hazards has been obtained from observations in the following circumstances.
1. Complications resulting from occupation, i.e. morbidity in radiologists, radiographers
etc.
2. A study of the radiotherapeutic side effects in patients.
3. Results of animal experiments.
4. Observations in survivors of atomic explosions.

**Radiation Hazards**    The possible effects may be classified as:
1. Latent, e.g. squamous cell carcinoma or leukaemia developing many years after exposure.
2. Genetic, e.g. sterility, repeated abortion or developmental abnormalities.
3. Immediate.
a) *General*
(i) Cerebral syndrome 5000r or more. Death occurs in one to two days from shock.
(ii) Gastrointestinal tract lesions after exposure of 800 – 5000r. Death occurs in about 10 days.
(iii) Bone marrow suppression can occur after exposure of less than 800r; death may occur in approximately 3 weeks.
b) *Local* (oral and para-oral structures)
(i)   Skin
(ii)  Oral mucous membrane
(iii) Salivary gland
(iv)  Teeth
(v)   Bone

*Skin*  1. Erythema begins in a few days after irradiation but fades quickly, only to reappear in 2 to 4 weeks. This fades slowly and may leave pigmentation; or the secondary erythema may be accompanied by marked oedema and desquamation resulting in denudation of the surface epithelium. Re-epithelialization occurs in 10 to 14 days. Early effects are caused by direct injury to cells and tissues. Late effects are caused by changes in vascular bed and intercellular material.
2. Sebaceous glandular activity is diminished, causing dry skin.
3. Epilation either temporary or permanent may be produced.
4. Sweat-glandular activity similarly disturbed causing dry and scaling skin.
5. Blood vessels superficially become telangiectatic or occluded — thickening of intima and thrombosis. Endophlebitis and phlebosclerosis may be particularly marked.

*Oral mucous membrane*  Same effects as on skin but with lower dosage of radiation and earlier onset.

*Salivary glands*  Xerostomia is the earliest and most universal of complaints and may begin within a week or two. The morphological changes seem unrelated to the physiological changes. However, there may be a decrease in the number of secretory granules in the acinar cells together with congestion, oedema and inflammatory cell infiltration.

*Teeth*  A. *Erupted teeth*
1. Enamel. Erupted teeth are often affected but lesions may not appear for several years after radiation. Destruction of tooth substance occurs resembling caries called 'radiation caries' located at the cervical area of teeth and sometimes causes amputation of tooth crown at its neck. Teeth are often friable and pieces break away.
2. Dentine. Impaired formation.
3. Pulp. Degeneration.
4. Gingivitis.
B. *Developing teeth*
1. Anodontia.
2. Hypoplasia and stunting of growth.
3. Delayed eruption.

*Bone*  Normal balance between bone formation and destruction is disturbed. General bone is decreased and localized osteoporosis may result in fracture. Bone is unable to react in normal fashion to infections because of:

1. Damage to vascular bed $\Big\}$ usually permanent
2. Damage to osteoblasts
Osteoradionecrosis can follow heavy irradiation of bone. Its main features are chronic, painful infection and necrosis together with sequestration. Three factors cause it:
(i) Radiation
(ii) Trauma
(iii) Infection
In one series 5 per cent of irradiated patients died of osteoradionecrosis without evidence of cancer.

*Preventive measures*    These should include a consideration of the following:
1. Patient.
2. Operator. The use of film badges.
3. Equipment.
4. Surgery design.

**Injuries, Fatigue and**    Injuries may be immediate or gradual and involve:
**Stress**    1. Hands.
2. Eyes.
3. Ears. Acoustic trauma depends on the age of the operator, susceptibility, time of exposure, volume and pitch of noise.
4. Musculo-skeletal deformities.
5. Other physical effects, e.g. varicose veins, haemorrhoids and pes planus.
6. Mental disorders. The suicide rate in the dental profession is known to be high.

# Chapter 15　Medico – Legal Aspects

There has been a steady increase in litigation over medical and dental treatment. Claims may be served under common law or various statutes, and the dentist may be requested to submit a report which can be used as evidence, and to act as a witness in court. A dentist who agrees to submit a report is entitled to a fee, and should consult his defence society.

It must be emphasized that a relevant history, correct clinical examination and results of investigations must lead to a completely impartial assessment.

Perhaps the commonest medico – legal problems are accident cases that are referred months later to an independent assessor. The assessor, having satisfied himself that he is willing to undertake the case, is sufficiently qualified and he is an impartial position, should report broadly as follows:

**History**　Accident. The date and time of injury, loss of consciousness, mode and cause of accident and any treatment priot to hospital admission should be included.

a) *Date and time of injury.* This will give some idea of how far advanced union should be for this particular case.

b) *Loss of consciousness.* The degree and duration and if it was anterograde or retrograde amnesia.

Remember to find out circumstances leading up to accident — alcohol, epilepsy, diabetes, stroke and heart attack are examples.

c) *Mode and cause of accident.* This may give the possible fracture lines — determined by (a) degree of force; (b) resistance to force (head fixed or not); (c) direction of force; (d) point of application; (e) size of object; (f) muscles attached.

d) *Treatment prior to admission to hospital.* Find out if patient had (a) antibiotics, (b) morphine, (c) anti-tetanus, (d) other medications.

*Hospital management.* A record of treatment before, during and after surgery should be obtained.

*Presenting complaints.* The patient may complain of altered appearance, difficulty in eating, swallowing and speaking, persistent pain, swelling and discharge. Changes in smell, sight, hearing, balance and facial sensation may also be presenting features. Finally, any relevant information from the medical, family and personal histories should be noted. Previous photographs and dental models of the patient can be useful.

**Examination**   The results of the examination of a soft or hard tissue lesion, extent of hyperaesthesia or anaesthesia, occlusal defects, swellings and neurological assessment, where indicated, should be included in the report.

**Investigations**   It may be necessary to undertake a number of investigations. These may include radiographs, smear and culture, haematology, aspiration and biopsy.

**Summary**   The essential feature should be impartiality. Only relevant facts should be reported and no attempt should be made to include opinions, prognoses and conclusions.